T0091487

NEUROLOGY AND NEUROSURGERY

200 SBAs for Medical Students

NEUROLOGY AND NEUROSURGERY

200 SBAs for Medical Students

Conor Gillespie
Ameer Khan

University of Liverpool, UK

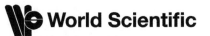
World Scientific

NEW JERSEY · LONDON · SINGAPORE · BEIJING · SHANGHAI · HONG KONG · TAIPEI · CHENNAI · TOKYO

Published by

World Scientific Publishing Co. Pte. Ltd.

5 Toh Tuck Link, Singapore 596224

USA office: 27 Warren Street, Suite 401-402, Hackensack, NJ 07601

UK office: 57 Shelton Street, Covent Garden, London WC2H 9HE

British Library Cataloguing-in-Publication Data
A catalogue record for this book is available from the British Library.

NEUROLOGY AND NEUROSURGERY
200 SBAs for Medical Students

ISBN 978-981-125-030-9 (hardcover)
ISBN 978-981-125-101-6 (paperback)
ISBN 978-981-125-031-6 (ebook for institutions)
ISBN 978-981-125-032-3 (ebook for individuals)

For any available supplementary material, please visit
https://www.worldscientific.com/worldscibooks/10.1142/12666#t=suppl

Printed in Singapore

Dedications

To Alex, Ben, and Sam, thank you for your unwavering support and friendship. Abed, I couldn't have wished for a better mentor. Natasha, thank you for helping me get through a difficult time. I'll always be grateful.

— Conor Gillespie

To my dearest Mum and Dad and all my family and friends who have pushed and supported me to get to this position in life.

— Ameer Khan

Foreword

This book presents a series of 200 questions covering neurology and neurosurgery topics for medical students taking their final exams. As clinical neuroscience can be a daunting topic for medical students, this book aims to cover all the important topics with a clear explanation of the correct answer to each question. The book was conceived and prepared by a dedicated medical student (Conor Gillespie) with input from other medical students, junior doctors, and consultants — all with the aim of making the book as relevant and as accessible as possible to those with 'neurophobia'. To this end the goal has been achieved, and this book should sit in every medical school library and medical student book shelf. We must remember that the people who gain the most from good clinical neuroscience knowledge are our patients.

— Professor Michael Jenkinson
Professor of Neurosurgery and Sir John Fisher / RCSEng Chair of Surgical Trials
University of Liverpool and The Walton Centre NHS Foundation Trust

Preface

The goal of this book is simple. Use this, and never have to worry about clinical neuro again. The Single Best Answer (SBAs) in this book are a mixture of core knowledge and challenging questions, all designed for medical students approaching the final years of their course. One of the most reported reasons why students find neuro difficult is its depth, so we have sought to ameliorate this problem with focused questions and unique 'one-sentence summaries' of each neuro condition containing almost all the vital information you need to know for the purposes of exams and being a good clinician, and nothing more. A shape system is also in place detailing which topics are essential for exams (circle), less essential (square), and for those hoping to distinguish themselves clinically (triangle).

My tip for the self-confessed neurophobe, who hopes that no questions on neurology or neurosurgery come up in exams, would be: just read this book; it has been tailored to this purpose.

The book has been divided into 5 question papers. The papers get progressively more difficult and incorporate some of the answers to the previous papers, ensuring dynamic ascertainment and aggregation of knowledge throughout.

Our advice is to go through the first paper and then the answers, as these come in useful for answering questions in the papers that follow, aiding memory recall. At the end of the book is a glossary of one-sentence summaries about each condition, which form the core essentials to be referred to.

There are a few things not covered in this book, namely ENT and neuroanatomy. A lot of books do neuroanatomy better than I ever could, and I've never really been sharp at ENT to be honest!

This book took forever and a day to finish, so I really hope you like it!

— Conor Gillespie

About the Authors

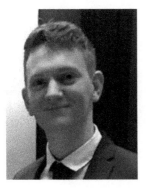

Conor Gillespie is a final year medical student at the University of Liverpool. He intercalated, completing an MPhil in Surgery and Oncology under Professor Michael Jenkinson at the University of Liverpool. His interests include clinical neurosciences, neuro-oncology, neurosurgery, and medical education. He is the recipient of a grant from the Wolfson foundation, a national award for intercalating students who excel academically. He was also awarded the Benjamin Ordman prize, given to the highest exam performance in the third year of medical school out of 290 students. He was the clinical and overall winner of the 2021 National Undergraduate Neuroanatomy Competition (NUNC).

Outside of medicine, Conor enjoys football and formula one. He is also passionate about mental health and community work.

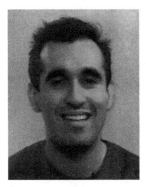

Ameer Khan is a final year medical student at the University of Liverpool. During his fourth year, he served as the BMA rep for Liverpool before being promoted to the regional north west committee. He is interested in Cardiology, general medicine, and medical education.

He is a coffee enthusiast, a big foodie, and an even bigger Liverpool FC fan.

List of Editors and Illustrators

Senior authors:

Rhys Davies MA BMBCh, PhD, FRCP
Consultant Neurologist and Honorary Senior Lecturer, The Walton Centre NHS Foundation Trust, Liverpool, UK

Viraj Bharambe BM BSc (Hons) MRCP
Neurology specialist registrar, The Walton Centre NHS Foundation Trust, Liverpool, UK

Benedict D. Michael MBChB, MRCP, PhD
Senior Clinician Scientist Fellow and Honorary Consultant Neurologist, University of Liverpool, Walton Centre NHS Foundation Trust, Liverpool, UK

Abdurrahman Islim MPhil, MBChB
Academic Foundation Doctor, Royal Liverpool and Broadgreen NHS Foundation Trust, Liverpool, UK

Ali Bakhsh MRCS, BMBS (dist), MSc, BSc (Hons), FHEA
Academic Clinical Fellow in Neurosurgery, the Walton Centre NHS Foundation Trust, Liverpool, UK

Christopher Paul Millward MRCS, MSc, MBBS, BSc
Neurosurgery Trainee, The Walton Centre NHS Foundation Trust, Liverpool, UK

Michael D. Jenkinson MBChB (Hons), PhD, FRCSEd (Neuro Surg)
Professor of Neurosurgery and Sir John Fisher / RCSEng Chair of Surgical Trials, University of Liverpool, The Walton Centre NHS Foundation Trust, Liverpool, UK

Chapter Editors and Reviewers

Practice paper 2: George E Richardson MRes (candidate), MBChB (candidate) and Mohammad A Mustafa MRes (candidate), MBChB (candidate)

Medical student, University of Liverpool, Liverpool, UK

Practice paper 3: Basel A Taweel MPhil (candidate), MBChB (candidate) and Khaleefa Al-Naham MBChB

Medical student, University of Liverpool, UK

Practice paper 4: Roshan K Babar MPhil (candidate), MBChB (candidate)

Medical student, University of Liverpool, UK

Practice paper 5: Ali Bakhsh MRCS, BMBS (dist), MSc, BSc (Hons), FHEA

Academic Clinical Fellow in Neurosurgery, the Walton Centre NHS Foundation Trust, Liverpool, UK

Acknowledgments

The authors would like to thank all of the brilliant staff at the Walton Centre NHS Foundation Trust — without their mentorship, inspiration and support, this book would not have been possible.

The front cover of this book was designed by rawpixel.com / Freepik.

Disclaimer

This book is for educational purposes only and should not be used to directly guide clinical practice. Many of the things reported in this book may change as guidelines evolve. If ever in doubt, please use your local trust/hospital guidelines.

Contents

Practice Paper 1

1. **Cushing's triad of raised intracranial pressure includes what?**

    A. Hypertension, tachycardia, irregular respiration

    B. Hypotension, bradycardia, tachypnoea

    C. Supranuclear gaze palsy, pseudo-argyll Robertson pupils, nystagmus

    D. Bradycardia, hypertension, irregular respiration

    E. Ptosis, miosis, facial anhidrosis

2. **A patient has recently been diagnosed as having a chronic subdural haematoma. What patient presentation would most likely represent this case?**

    A. 23-year-old male who sustained an injury whilst playing cricket. He lost consciousness initially, recovered quickly, before deteriorating again an hour later.

    B. 65-year-old with chronic alcohol dependency presents to the emergency department 4 hours after falling down a flight of stairs. On examination, she has 3/5 power on the left-hand side.

    C. 28-year-old male presents with sudden onset headache that occurred during sexual intercourse with his partner. On examination, he has marked neck stiffness.

    D. 85-year-old female presents to the A&E accompanied by her daughter. For the last two weeks she has been intermittently confused and her daughter does not know why. She has diabetic peripheral neuropathy and atrial fibrillation, and takes warfarin for this.

    E. 55-year-old male presents with a 2-hour history of sudden onset left arm weakness that occurred whilst watching TV.

3. **A 63-year-old patient presents to the hospital's A&E department after tripping over one of the plants in his garden and hitting his head on a plant pot. He is normally fit and well with no medical history. He did not lose consciousness and has a GCS of 15 on examination, in addition to bruising behind the mastoid process and some clear nasal discharge. He is now 2 hours post-injury. His mini mental state examination is normal and he reports feeling well. What is the most appropriate management for this patient in the A&E?**

    A. 300mg Aspirin, bleep stroke consultant

    B. Refer for neurosurgery outpatient appointment

    C. No requirement for CT head scan, can be discharged with safety netting

    D. CT head scan within the next 8 hours

    E. CT head scan within 1 hour

4.   A 22-year-old female presents with worsening headaches for 3 months. These headaches are worse when she gets out of bed, bends over, or coughs. She also complains of reduced visual quality. She has a recent diagnosis of polycystic ovarian syndrome and has gained around 2 stone (13 kg) in the past year — her body mass index is now 38. On examination you find papilloedema and no other deficits, but her CT head scan results are normal. What is the most likely diagnosis?

A.   Tension headache

B.   Glioblastoma

C.   Idiopathic intracranial hypertension

D.   Cavernous sinus thrombosis

E.   Chronic subdural haematoma

5.   Janice, an 82-year-old female, presents with sudden onset left-sided weakness whilst watching TV. Her husband also noted that her speech is slurred. She is normally fit and well and does not take any medications. She is seen by the stroke consultant on-call and diagnosed with a suspected acute right total anterior circulatory stroke, and after a normal CT head scan undergoes thrombolysis 4 hours after symptom onset. 3 hours later, she appears drowsy and suddenly becomes unresponsive. What is the most likely diagnosis?

A.   Overuse of opiate medication

B.   Malignant middle cerebral artery syndrome

C.   Subarachnoid haemorrhage

D.   Haemorrhagic transformation of infarct

E.   Hypoglycaemia

6.   A 28-year-old male who is normally fit and well presents in a dishevelled state. His wife tells you he reported headaches for the past week, with the worst ones occurring first thing in the morning. In the past 4 days, he has developed a fever of 39.5°C and left leg weakness, and he is confused. His past history is unremarkable apart from having occasional migraines, and he recovered from an episode of sinusitis 2 weeks ago. He has not travelled abroad recently and does not use intravenous drugs. A CT scan shows a round, ring-enhancing lesion in the frontal lobe. What is the most likely diagnosis?

A.   Encephalitis

B.   Meningitis

C.   Central nervous system lymphoma

D.   Cerebral abscess

E.   Tuberculosis

7.   A 65-year-old male presents to the general practitioner with bilateral leg pains. He has a 15-year history of poorly controlled type 2 diabetes and benign prostatic hyperplasia. He describes the pain as 'dull' and 'like an electric shock', and it is stopping him from sleeping. Which of the following agents should be avoided when treating this man's pain?

   A.   Pregabalin

   B.   Duloxetine

▲ C.   Amitriptyline

   D.   Gabapentin

   E.   Paracetamol

8.   A 23-year-old male presents to the A&E after an assault. On examination, he opens his eyes when a trapezius squeeze is applied, and he is groaning but not formulating any words. When you apply a pain stimulus to his shoulder, he pulls his limb away from the stimulus. What is the likely score on the patient's Glasgow Coma Scale?

   A.   6

   B.   7

● C.   8

   D.   9

   E.   10

9.   A patient is referred to a neurologist outpatient clinic with a suspected diagnosis of Horner's syndrome. What describes the classical features of this syndrome?

   A.   Ptosis, mydriasis, exophthalmos

   B.   Ptosis, miosis, facial anhydrosis, enophthalmos

● C.   Miosis, mydriasis, exophthalmos

   D.   Ataxia, ophthalmoplegia, confusion

   E.   Headache, fever, altered consciousness

10.   A 36-year-old female attends the A&E department with a 2-hour history of sudden onset headache, which she describes as like 'being hit over the head with a baseball bat'. The on-call neurologist suspects a subarachnoid haemorrhage. Her CT head scan at 2 hours after onset is reported as normal by a consultant radiologist. What is the most appropriate next investigation to undertake?

A.   CT angiography at 24 hours

B.   Repeat CT head scan at 12 hours

C.   Repeat CT head scan at 2 hours

D.   Lumbar puncture immediately

E.   Lumbar puncture at 12 hours

11.   A 65-year-old retired army sergeant attends the GP with his wife. She reports that for the past two years, he has appeared lethargic, lost significant muscle mass compared to his army days, and has had problems swallowing food. On examination, the patient appears emaciated with widespread muscle wasting, and you note the presence of fasciculations on his tongue. His reflexes are weak, he has a positive Babinski sign in both legs, and his sensory function is intact. What is the most likely diagnosis?

A.   Amyotrophic lateral sclerosis

B.   Parkinson's disease

C.   Huntington's disease

D.   Multiple sclerosis

E.   Duchenne's muscular dystrophy

12.   A patient is referred to a neurology outpatient clinic with memory loss. After taking his history, the doctor suspects normal pressure hydrocephalus. What is the triad associated with this presentation of symptoms?

A.   Personality change, frequent falls, leg weakness

B.   Dementia, impotence, fluctuating consciousness

C.   Dementia, dysarthria, dysphonia

D.   Urinary incontinence, gait ataxia, dementia

E.   Urinary frequency, dementia, frequent falls

13.   A 57-year-old male is diagnosed with a brain tumour after presenting with a 2-month history of headaches. The tumour is removed and diagnosed as a brain metastasis. Which cancer is the most common primary source of brain metastases?

   A.   Breast
   B.   Melanoma
   C.   Kidney
   D.   Lung
   E.   Liver

14.   Which of the following is NOT an absolute contraindication to having a lumbar puncture?

   A.   Glasgow Coma Scale of 8
   B.   Heart rate of 45 and blood pressure of 180/105, five minutes before the lumbar puncture
   C.   Papilloedema
   D.   Cardio or respiratory instability
   E.   Headache

15.   A 23-year-old male patient attends an epilepsy review, diagnosed after having two tonic-clonic seizures one year ago. While his seizures have stopped since commencing medication, he complains of unintentional weight gain of 8kg since starting them. Which anti-convulsant medication is most associated with weight gain?

   A.   Sodium valproate
   B.   Levetiracetam (Keppra®)
   C.   Lamotrigine
   D.   Carbamazepine
   E.   Phenytoin

16.   A 28-year-old male accountant attends his GP with troublesome right-sided headaches for the past 6 months. He describes experiencing up to two episodes of headache each day, always around 8pm. The episodes last for 2 hours each time. When he has an episode, it is excruciatingly painful, and he reports having to walk around in circles until the pain subsides. On occasion, he reports excessive tearing from the right eye. Neurological examination is normal, there is no neck stiffness, and ophthalmoscopy is normal. Which of the following is the most likely diagnosis?

A.   Migraine

B.   Tension headache

C.   Cluster headache

D.   Space-occupying lesion

E.   Medication overuse headache

17.   A 31-year-old female dental nurse attends the GP. For the past two weeks she has been extremely troubled by intense left-sided facial pain. The pain originates from the angle of her jaw and travels to the corner of her mouth, and she describes the pain as 'like little electric shocks'. She has noticed that area of her face is now extremely sensitive, and the pain can be brought on by touching the area. She is normally fit and well, has no allergies, and does not take any medication. The week before, she went for a check-up with her dentist, who gave her the all-clear. What is the most likely diagnosis?

A.   Temporomandibular joint dysfunction

B.   Paroxysmal hemicrania

C.   Multiple sclerosis

D.   Dental-related pain

E.   Trigeminal neuralgia

18.   For the previous question (17), assuming there are no contraindications, what is the first line treatment to start the patient on?

A.   Lithium

B.   Propranolol

C.   Primidone

D.   Carbamazepine

E.   Sodium valproate

19.   A 73-year-old male presents to the A&E department. 4 hours earlier, his wife
       noticed that, while watching TV, his speech suddenly became slurred and he could
       not move his left arm. He has a past medical history of hypertension and type 2
       diabetes, for which he currently takes ramipril and gliclazide respectively. An
       acute stroke is suspected. What is the most appropriate initial investigation for
       this patient (whilst in the emergency department)?

       A.   Immediate contrast CT head scan

       B.   Immediate non-contrast CT head scan

   C.   Urgent MRI brain scan

       D.   Urine dipstick

       E.   Capillary blood glucose

20.   The concerned parents of a 9-month-old baby bring him to a GP. Over the past
       2 months, they describe the child as having frequent episodes of flexing his arms
       towards his chest before straightening them out, whilst drawing his knees up to
       his chest. On examination, he cannot sit upright, has poor head control, and does
       not babble or say any words. They had attended a GP appointment 3 months ago
       and the locum GP diagnosed him with colic, but this has not resolved. What is
       the most likely diagnosis?

       A.   Infantile spasms (West syndrome)

       B.   Absence seizures

       C.   Benign Rolandic epilepsy

       D.   Juvenile myoclonic epilepsy

       E.   Panayiotopoulos syndrome

21.   You are an F1 doctor doing a ward round on a stroke ward. The stroke consultant
       asks the next patient, who is recovering from a left partial anterior circulation
       stroke, how he is doing. The patient replies, 'Nice very breakfast my own horse
       but then spaceships purple today'. What best describes the patient's speech issue?

       A.   Broca's aphasia

       B.   Wernicke's aphasia

       C.   Conduction aphasia

       D.   Dysarthria

       E.   Dysphagia

22. Which of the following is NOT a risk factor for Carpal tunnel syndrome?

A. Female gender

B. Pregnancy

C. Multiple sclerosis

D. Rheumatoid arthritis

E. Hypothyroidism

23. You see a 48-year-old homeless male with a history of alcohol misuse and chronic pancreatitis, who was brought into the ward after being found confused by a friend. His friend reports that he had not eaten or drank anything for days and is confused and struggling to walk. You suspect that he may have Wernicke's encephalopathy. What is the triad for Wernicke's encephalopathy?

A. Confusion, dysarthria, dysphasia

B. Confusion, ataxia, ophthalmoplegia

C. Nystagmus, ataxia, ophthalmoplegia

D. Confusion, vomiting, dementia

E. Diarrhoea, dermatitis, dementia

24. A 12-year-old boy is accompanied by his mother to a GP appointment, and he states that his legs feel tired after walking. He was adopted as a young child and has no other past medical history. On examination, the patient appears to have grossly misshapen feet in a concave appearance, hammer toes, and some evidence of distal muscle wasting of the leg. The patient otherwise appears well. What is the inheritance pattern of the most likely diagnosis?

A. Autosomal dominant

B. Autosomal recessive

C. X-linked recessive

D. X-linked dominant

E. Mitochondrial

25.   You are in clinic with a neurology registrar, during which he gets bored and decides to grill you on your neuroanatomy. He asks which dermatome supplies the ventral aspect of the little finger. What is the correct answer?

A. C6

B. C7

C. C8

D. T1

E. T2

26.   In the same clinic with the neurology registrar, you examine a patient with suspected degenerative cervical myelopathy, referred for her first specialist appointment by her GP. The neurology registrar holds the patient's hand and flicks the nail of the middle finger, and you notice the patient's thumb and index finger flex spontaneously. What is the sign being elicited?

A. Babinski's sign

B. Hoover's sign

C. Hoffman's sign

D. Brudzinski's sign

E. Lhermitte's sign

27.   You are a final year medical student with your own clinic in a GP surgery. Your next patient is a 70-year-old male. For the past 6 months, he appears to have slowed down, taking much longer to get dressed in the morning and return from the shops. On further questioning, he trivially reports losing his sense of smell 2 years ago, and his handwriting appears much smaller than it used to. On examination, you notice a 3–5 Hz tremor that disappears when he moves his arm, and he has a fixed, limited facial expression. What is the most likely diagnosis?

A. Multiple systems atrophy

B. Motor neurone disease

C. Idiopathic Parkinson's disease

D. Corticobasal degeneration

E. Frontotemporal dementia

28. **Which of the following is a feature of an upper motor neuron lesion?**

    A. Muscle wasting

    B. Fasciculations

    C. Diminished or absent reflexes

    D. Positive Babinski's sign

    E. Hypotonia

29. **A 75-year-old female is brought by ambulance to the A&E after falling down a flight of stairs while celebrating a friend's diamond wedding anniversary. She has a past history of alcohol misuse and atrial fibrillation, for which she takes apixaban 5mg once daily. Her only other regular medication is atorvastatin 20mg once nightly. She appears confused, and the paramedics hand over that she has a GCS of 10. A CT head scan shows a hyperdense, crescent-shaped opacity that crosses suture lines with no skull fractures. What is the most likely diagnosis?**

    A. Acute extradural haematoma

    B. Acute subdural haematoma

    C. Chronic subdural haematoma

    D. Basal skull fracture

    E. Pneumocephalus

30. **A 2-week-old baby is referred to the neurosurgical team after being found to have a rapidly enlarging head circumference, which is now measured to be in the 98th percentile. She was born prematurely at 32 weeks due to foetal distress and suffered an intraventricular haemorrhage at 2 days old. The paediatric neurosurgery registrar suspects hydrocephalus. Which of the following examination signs will NOT be present?**

    A. Enlarged head circumference

    B. Dilated scalp veins

    C. Sun setting of eyes

    D. Microcephaly

    E. Bulging anterior fontanelle

31.   Ben, a 22-year-old medical student, attends his GP in a very concerned state. For
        the past 2 months, he has complained of feeling dizzy, often after standing up.
        He is very worried that he might have an arrythmia, and he has read all about
        them as part of his studies. His lying and standing blood pressure measurements
        are within normal range, and his 7-day ambulatory ECG reveals 8 ectopic beats
        along with sinus rhythm. He does not take these results well. In his notes over the
        last 4 years, he has undergone checks at a genitourinary medicine clinic with an
        eventual diagnosis of non-gonococcal urethritis, was investigated for dysphagia
        with no pathological cause found, and had a benign skin mole removed after
        expressing concern. What is the most likely diagnosis?

        A.   Somatisation disorder

        B.   Arrythmia

    ▲   C.   Munchausen's syndrome

        D.   Hypochondriac disorder

        E.   Acquired immunodeficiency

32.   Mohammed, a 72-year-old retired pilot presents to his GP with a sudden onset
        of back pain for the last 2 days. He describes having a pain 'like an elastic band'
        in his upper abdomen and back for 8 weeks, but did not seek treatment because
        he 'did not want to be a bother'. He is normally fully mobile, but for the last 2
        days has found getting about the house difficult. He has no urinary incontinence.
        He has a past history of prostate cancer, and he underwent radiotherapy 12 months
        ago for a recurrence. On examination, he has MRC grade 2/5 power in both lower
        limbs. What is the most appropriate immediate management for this patient?

        A.   Immediate neurosurgical decompression

        B.   Urgent oncology referral for radiotherapy

    ●   C.   Position the patient upright

        D.   Give the patient dexamethasone 16mg

        E.   Urgent MRI scan (within 12 hours)

33.   A patient is brought into the A&E after suffering a stab wound to the back during
        a fight in the city centre. On examination, the patient has considerable neurological
        deficits and a right-sided stab wound. The consultant suspects a diagnosis of
        Brown-Séquard syndrome. What examination findings would you expect?

        A.   Right-sided loss of pain and temperature, left-sided weakness

        B.   Right-sided leg weakness and loss of pain and temperature, left-sided loss of
             proprioception and vibration

    ●   C.   Right-sided weakness, right-sided loss of pain and temperature

        D.   Left-sided loss of pain and temperature only

        E.   Right-sided leg weakness and loss of vibration and proprioception, left-sided loss
             of pain and temperature

34.   You are on rotation at a medical ward when one of the senior house officers
        suggests that you examine the eyes of a 65-year-old patient. On examination, the
        patient's right eyelid is significantly lower than that of the left, and his right pupil
        is fixed and unreactive to light. When the patient is asked to look straight ahead,
        the left eye looks forward, but the right eye appears located in the right lower
        quadrant of the eye. Which cranial nerve is affected?

        A.   Second cranial nerve (optic)

        B.   Third cranial nerve (oculomotor)

        C.   Fourth cranial nerve (trochlear)

        D.   Fifth cranial nerve (trigeminal)

        E.   Sixth cranial nerve (abducens)

35.   Kyle, a 12-year-old boy, is brought to his GP by his concerned parents. They have
        noticed that over the last few months, his performance in school has steadily
        declined. He used to be at the top of his class for mathematics, but now he struggles
        to do basic sums. His mum reports that he forgot the names of his friends when
        they came over to play football last week, and he has become a lot more quiet. On
        examination, the patient has a resting tremor, and you note the presence of a
        golden-brown ring around his eyes. He is normally fit and well, and there is no
        family history. What is the most likely diagnosis?

        A.   Inherited Parkinson's disease

        B.   Subacute sclerosing panencephalitis

        C.   Wilson's disease

        D.   Huntington's

        E.   Tertiary syphilis

36.   Reginald, a 70-year-old retired navy captain, comes to see his GP. He apologises,
        saying his wife made him come in. In the last 6 months, his shoe size has gone up
        three sizes, and he has noticed his wedding ring no longer fits on his finger, but
        he denies recent weight gain. His past medical history includes hypertension
        resistant to 3 anti-hypertensive medications and bilateral carpal tunnel syndrome.
        On examination, you note prognathism and a very large tongue. What is the most
        likely visual deficit you will see on examination?

        A.   Unilateral blindness

        B.   Bitemporal superior hemianopia

        C.   Bitemporal inferior hemianopia

        D.   Left-sided homonymous hemianopia

        E.   Bilateral homonymous hemianopia with macular sparing

37.   A 55-year-old man has been at the intensive care unit for the past 6 weeks after being involved in a high-speed motor vehicle accident. He was not wearing a seatbelt and he had a GCS of 3 at the scene. His recovery has been slow and he is unable to be taken off the ventilator. A CT head scan shows small punctate contusions but is otherwise normal. What is the most likely diagnosis?

A.   Extradural haematoma

B.   Coning due to raised intracranial pressure

C.   Hydrocephalus

D.   Diffuse axonal Injury

E.   Subdural haematoma

38.   You are in the A&E as a foundation doctor and the consultant shows you the image below. What is the most likely diagnosis?

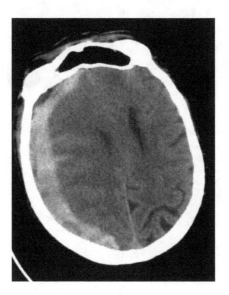

*With permission from Dr Christopher McLeavy, Royal Liverpool and Broadgreen University Hospitals NHS Trust, UK

A.   Hydrocephalus

B.   Acute extradural haematoma

C.   Normal scan

D.   Subarachnoid haemorrhage

E.   Acute subdural haematoma

39.   On the same shift, another F1 approaches you and asks you to help them interpret another scan. This patient was admitted to their acute medical ward after being found unresponsive at home, and he has a significant focal neurological deficit. Based on their CT scan taken 2 hours ago, what is the most likely diagnosis?

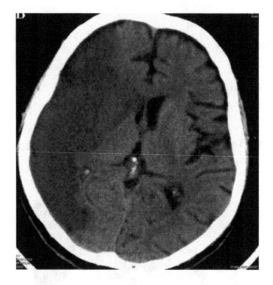

*With permission from Dr Christopher McLeavy, Royal Liverpool and Broadgreen University Hospitals NHS Trust, UK

A.   Chronic subdural haematoma

B.   Middle cerebral artery infarction

C.   Diffuse axonal injury

D.   Hydrocephalus

E.   Acute extradural haematoma

40. A 38-year-old scaffolder attends the A&E department after an accident at work where 12 bricks fell on his neck, causing it to bend downwards. He noticed immediate weakness and altered sensation afterwards. On examination, he has MRC grade 2/5 power in both legs, but grade 4/5 power in both arms and grade 5/5 power in the rest of the upper limbs. He cannot feel a pinprick on his legs, but can recognise when a tuning fork is placed on them. What is the most likely diagnosis?

    A. Anterior cord syndrome

    B. Central cord syndrome

    C. Syringomyelia

    D. Brown-Sequard syndrome

    E. Spinal shock

Practice Paper 2

1.   Mary is a 78-year-old female who was referred by her GP to the movement disorders clinic with a suspected diagnosis of Parkinson's. She has noticed that, over the last 6 months, she has developed a resting tremor that improves with movement, and she has slowed significantly. On taking a more detailed history, she reports that before her symptoms started, she began suffering from frequent falls and now uses a wheelchair to prevent them from happening. On examination, she has limited eye movements and cannot move them upwards, as well as a fixed facial expression with the appearance of looking surprised. What is the most likely diagnosis?

     A.   Idiopathic Parkinson's disease

     B.   Corticobasal degeneration

      C.   Multiple systems atrophy

     D.   Progressive supranuclear palsy

     E.   Drug-induced parkinsonism

2.   Annie is a 36-year-old Caucasian female who has presented to her GP. Last week, she noticed a gradual onset of left eye pain with associated blurred vision, which has now thankfully settled down. She has a past medical history of hypothyroidism and depression, and is taking thyroxine and sertraline for these respectively. She reports no headaches or previous episodes and no other symptoms, although she does report having a sudden onset of numbness with mild weakness of her right leg for 2 days in the previous year. On examination, her vision is normal. What is the most likely diagnosis?

     A.   Amaurosis fugax

     B.   Primary angle glaucoma

     C.   Multiple sclerosis

     D.   Conversion disorder

     E.   Space-occupying lesion

3.   Mahmood is a 65-year-old male with a new diagnosis of amyotrophic lateral sclerosis by his neurologist. The prognosis and clinical course have been explained to him. He asks the neurologist if there are any medications that may help him live longer, as his daughter is currently a third year medical student and it would mean everything to him to see her graduate. What drug improves survival in patients with his condition?

A.   Riluzole

B.   Dexamethasone

C.   Prednisolone

D.   Tetrabenazine

E.   Natalizumab

4.   Gerry, a 34-year-old male patient at your GP clinic, has recently been diagnosed with Huntington's. The inherited nature of the condition has been explained to him. After being quite reserved throughout the consultation, he tells you that his wife is currently 28 weeks pregnant with their first child, a baby boy. He is worried about passing the condition on to his son and asks you what his son's chances are of inheriting the disease. His wife is not affected by the condition. What do you tell him?

A.   Impossible to determine without further family history

B.   25%

C.   50%

D.   100%

E.   0%

5.   A 25-year-old PhD student attends the epilepsy clinic after having a suspected first seizure. This was noticed by her partner, who describes finding her 'shaking her limbs and then going stiff' for ten minutes in the morning. The episode resolved spontaneously, and she had no urinary or faecal incontinence, bit the centre of her tongue, and was noticeably tearful immediately afterwards. He describes her eyes as being clenched shut during the episode. She has no past medical history, but reports being 'stressed out' as her PhD thesis is due next week. What is the most likely diagnosis?

A.   Generalised tonic-clonic seizure

B.   Non-epileptic attack disorder

C.   Conversion disorder

D.   Munchausen's syndrome

E.   Status epilepticus

6.   As an F2 doctor at work on Saturday, you are bleeped to see to an emergency at one of the wards. There, you find a worried nurse who explains that the patient is a 53-year-old male who underwent surgery to remove a brain tumour and has been fitting for the last 10 minutes. The nurse has secured his airway and is giving high flow oxygen via a non-rebreathe mask, and the patient is fitting continuously. You note a pink cannula located on the dorsum of the wrist placed by the anaesthetic team yesterday. After calling for help, what is your next immediate management?

   A.   Call the anaesthetic team for immediate support before commencing any management
   B.   Give IV phenytoin 15–25 mg/kg after setting up a large bore cannula
   C.   Give rectal diazepam 10 mg
   D.   Give IV lorazepam 4 mg
   E.   Wait another 20 minutes before intervening

7.   You are in a GP and your next patient is a 28-year-old female who is 12 weeks pregnant. For the past 6 weeks, she has been troubled by intense headaches. They happen once every few days and are dull and achy in nature. During an episode, she lies still and tries to go into a dark room, which sometimes helps. There are no associated visual disturbances and her blood pressure on examination is normal. The headaches impact her work as a primary school teacher and she is desperate to resolve them. Apart from well-controlled asthma with a salbutamol inhaler, she is well. What medication would you offer her to prevent her headaches?

   A.   Propranolol
   B.   Topiramate
   C.   Amitriptyline
   D.   Metoclopramide
   E.   Codeine phosphate

8.   You are the GP of Jean, a 78-year-old retired teacher from Wales. One day, she comes to you with a 2-week history of troublesome headache. The headache presented over a few days and is 8/10 in intensity. She also describes feeling tired and weak during the same period. She has noticed that the pain is brought on by combing her hair, and she has had some difficulty chewing foods which she thinks is unrelated. Bloods have already been taken and sent off to test for markers that would support the diagnosis. What is the most appropriate management step?

   A.   Wait for blood tests to come back before deciding on management
   B.   Urgent rheumatology referral
   C.   Book an urgent MRI brain scan
   D.   Start prednisolone 60–80 mg
   E.   Start prednisolone 15–20 mg

9.   A 35-year-old female patient presents to the neurology clinic. For the past 6 months, she has been feeling extremely tired and weak, most often at the end of her long day working as an accountant. She also complains of double vision, which occurs exclusively in the evenings. She had seen an optometrist who ruled out ophthalmological causes. On examination, she has MRC grade 5 power throughout initially; however, after flexing her arm 3 times, her power reduces to MRC grade 3. What is the most likely diagnosis?

A.   Myaesthenia gravis

B.   Lambert-Eaton myaesthenic syndrome

C.   Multiple sclerosis

D.   Amyotrophic lateral sclerosis

E.   Polymyalgia rheumatica

10.   You are in the A&E as a medical student and you see the consultant rush to a new patient in triage, thought to be having an acute stroke. While the patient is getting their CT scan, the registrar asks you, how long, after symptom onset, are patients eligible to receive thrombolysis and thrombectomy, respectively. What would the answer be?

A.   3 hours for thrombolysis, 6 hours for thrombectomy

B.   4.5 hours for thrombolysis, 18 hours for thrombectomy

C.   4.5 hours for thrombolysis, 6 hours for thrombectomy

D.   6 hours for thrombolysis, 24 hours for thrombectomy

E.   4.5 hours for thrombolysis, thrombectomy no longer recommended in stroke

11.   You are shadowing doctors as part of the acute medical unit ward round and come across the same patient you saw in the A&E the previous day (Question 10). The patient was not eligible for thrombolysis and suffered a large stroke. On examination, the patient's speech is slurred, and they appear frustrated when trying to answer the consultant's questions. They have a dense hemiplegia affecting the left-hand side of their whole body, and the consultant notes left-sided homonymous hemianopia on examination. According to the Bamford classification, what type of stroke do they have?

A.   Left total anterior circulatory stroke

B.   Right total anterior circulatory stroke

C.   Left partial anterior circulatory stroke

D.   Right partial anterior circulatory stroke

E.   Lacunar stroke

12.   A 25-year-old male railway engineer attends a GP surgery with his concerned parents. 8 weeks ago, he was working on the tracks when part of the track flew up and hit him on the head. Before the accident, he was very mild mannered, but since then he has become more aggressive, been in several bar fights, and lost ten thousand pounds of savings on slot machines. The patient does not appear concerned, swearing excessively throughout the consultation and demanding that he be allowed to leave as 'there is nothing wrong with me'. Which part of the brain is most likely affected?

A.   Global brain dysfunction

B.   Frontal lobe

C.   Parietal lobe

D.   Temporal lobe

E.   Occipital lobe

13.   An 82-year-old male sheepishly walks into a memory clinic with his wife. She is concerned about his memory, which has gradually declined over the past 2 years. He was an avid solver of newspaper crossword puzzles for many years, but now he cannot come up with a single answer. She has also noticed that, occasionally at night, he fails to recognise who she is even though they have been married for 50 years. He has worked as a bus driver all his life and is fit and well. On examination, he makes an active effort to address all questions asked, and his Montreal Cognitive Assessment score is 17/30. What is the most likely diagnosis?

A.   Mild cognitive impairment

B.   Depressive pseudodementia

C.   Alzheimer's disease

D.   Vascular dementia

E.   Frontotemporal dementia

14.   A 23-year-old male presents to the emergency department complaining of limb weakness starting with his legs, which has now moved up to his knee. He is very worried as the weakness has been getting worse since it started 10 days ago. Other than an episode of bad food poisoning 2 weeks ago after a 'dodgy takeaway', he is normally fit and well. Examination reveals MRC grade 2/5 power in both lower limbs, and reflexes are absent. What is the most likely diagnosis?

A.   Peripheral neuropathy

B.   Charcot-Marie-Tooth disease

C.   Space-occupying lesion

D.   Guillain-Barré syndrome

E.   Brown-Sequard syndrome

15.   You are in your final year OSCE assessment and have been asked to carry out a
        neurological motor examination. The patient's right side has normal power, but
        both the left arm and leg are weak. The patient cannot raise their arm or leg when
        asked to, but there is a flicker of contraction and the patient can flex the arm and
        leg when both are placed flat on the examination couch. The examiner asks you:
        What MRC grade power does this patient have on the left side?

        A.   Grade 5
        B.   Grade 4
        C.   Grade 3
        D.   Grade 2
        E.   Grade 1

16.   A 28-year-old female attends the neuro-ophthalmology clinic over an abnormality
        found during a routine eye test by her optician. She is asymptomatic. On
        examination, the right pupil is dilated and does not respond to the light reflex,
        but responds slowly to accommodation. Her eye movements are normal and there
        is no ptosis. The only other notable finding on examination is absent knee and
        ankle jerks. What is the most likely diagnosis?

        A.   Relative afferent pupillary defect
        B.   Holmes-Adie pupil
        C.   Argyll Robertson pupil
        D.   Vitamin B12 deficiency
        E.   Third cranial nerve palsy

17.   A 32-year-old male patient has a recent diagnosis of Creutzfeldt-Jakob disease
        and is seeing a neurologist. He complains of odd movements and describes them
        as sudden and uncontrollable electric shock-like jerks of his arm that last a second
        or two before resolving. He describes not experiencing restlessness. What
        movement disorder is he describing?

        A.   Dystonia
        B.   Akathisia
        C.   Tardive dyskinesia
        D.   Hemiballismus
        E.   Myoclonus

18.   An 18-year-old male from a travelling family presents to his local GP. For years, his parents have noticed irregular lumps throughout his whole body, but did not seek medical attention as he was asymptomatic and is otherwise well. On examination, he has several bumpy lesions occupying a dermatomal pattern in his upper limbs, strange freckles over his axilla, and a series of light, brown macules on his lower back. What is the most likely diagnosis?

A.   Tuberous sclerosis

B.   Sturge-Weber syndrome

C.   Neurofibromatosis type 1

D.   Neurofibromatosis type 2

E.   Adenoma sebaceum

19.   Whilst in clinic examining a patient with intractable vomiting, the consultant decides to test your anatomy and asks: in what region of the brain is the vomiting centre located?

A.   Midbrain

B.   Pons

C.   Medulla

D.   Area postrema

E.   Cerebrum

20.   A 19-year-old male is brought to the emergency department with a reduced consciousness level. He was playing cricket when a wayward ball struck him in the side of the head. His friend reports that he 'was out' for a few minutes but quickly regained consciousness, seemed fine and continued playing, until he collapsed 30 minutes later. His current GCS is 9. What is the most likely diagnosis?

A.   Acute subdural haematoma

B.   Acute extradural haematoma

C.   Post-concussion syndrome

D.   Subarachnoid haemorrhage

E.   Malignant MCA infarction

21.   Adel, a 54-year-old male, attends the neurosurgical clinic after an incidental mass was found during an MRI brain scan as part of a private health check. He is asymptomatic. The consultant explains to you that it is likely a tumour, located on the parietal convexity, with no brain invasion. The tumour is spherical and calcified. What is the most likely cause of his lesion?

A. Gliosis from previous surgery

B. Glioblastoma

C. Astrocytoma

D. Meningioma

E. Medulloblastoma

22.   A 35-year-old female attends the emergency department after experiencing a sudden onset of headache whilst having sexual intercourse with her husband. The pain is 10/10 in severity, and she describes it as 'like being hit over the head with a cricket bat' and it came on suddenly over 2–3 minutes. She has a past medical history of hypertension and currently takes amlodipine but nothing else. On examination, she has marked neck stiffness and is in considerable pain. What is the most likely diagnosis?

A. Meningitis

B. Encephalitis

C. Post-coital headache

D. Subarachnoid haemorrhage

E. Benign thunderclap headache

23.   Oliver, a 61-year-old semi-retired neurologist, comes to see you. He has been struggling over the past few months to use both his hands. He finds it difficult to do his buttons up in the morning, and finds it even harder to type up patient notes on the ward computers. He also says that the strength in his arms is 'a lot less than it used to be'. On examination, there is reduced power in the upper arms and muscles of the hand, and there is a positive Hoffman's sign. What is the most likely diagnosis?

A. Degenerative cervical myelopathy

B. Motor neurone disease

C. Primary lateral sclerosis

D. Lumbar radiculopathy

E. Multiple sclerosis

24.   Jennie, an 82-year-old female, visits the GP for her first appointment in ten years
        (she 'doesn't like to be a bother'). Over the last 24 hours, she has been troubled
        by terrible back pain, which came on without any trigger. Since then, she reports
        leg weakness and could not get out of her chair this morning, so she asks the GP
        for her first appointment in ten years. She reluctantly admits that she has had 'a
        few accidents' with her bowels and urine over the same period. On examination,
        she has reduced power in the legs and cannot feel any pinprick sensation in the
        peri-anal area. What is the most likely diagnosis?

        A.   Lumbar disc prolapse

        B.   Malignancy

    ●   C.   Cauda equina syndrome

        D.   Osteoporotic vertebral fracture

        E.   Urinary tract infection

25.   A 53-year-old male who has a known diagnosis of glioblastoma and is being
        managed with the best supportive care presents to the A&E department, acutely
        unwell with a reduced consciousness level. He was found by his ex-wife, and you
        have little history. On examination, his GCS is 8, breathing is regular, right pupil
        is fixed, dilated and unresponsive to light, and entire left-hand side is affected by
        a dense hemiparesis. What complication has the patient developed?

        A.   Tonsillar herniation

        B.   Subfalcine herniation

    ▲   C.   Hydrocephalus

        D.   Uncal (transtentorial) herniation

        E.   New onset stroke

26.   A 27-year-old female who is recovering from a bad episode of sinusitis presents
        to the A&E with painful eye movements and double vision. She is normally fit
        and well. On examination, there is significant eyeball protrusion and oedema
        surrounding both eyes. She has loss of forehead sensation bilaterally, and
        ophthalmoscopy reveals papilloedema. What is the most likely diagnosis?

        A.   Pituitary apoplexy

        B.   Cavernous sinus thrombosis

    ■   C.   Intracerebral malignancy

        D.   Idiopathic intracranial hypertension

        E.   Posterior communicating artery aneurysm

27. A 45-year-old male security guard collapsed at work and was brought to the A&E. He had complained to his colleagues of headaches that are most severe in the morning over the last 3 months as well as occasional double vision, but was determined to 'soldier on' and not seek medical advice. An emergency CT scan identifies a suspicious mass lesion in the frontal lobe with very prominent oedema around the mass. What medication should be given to reduce the oedema and help with his symptoms?

A. Nimodipine

B. Morphine sulphate

C. Dexamethasone

D. Mannitol

E. Acetazolamide

28. A 52-year-old male is brought into the emergency department by his partner, who is concerned about his behaviour. For the past 2 months his memory has declined significantly and he has forgotten to pay his bills, become very 'amped up' lately — sleeping for only 2 hours a night — and become unsteady on his feet. He has no prior history of mental health problems, although he had a stroke ten years ago and a sudden widespread body rash that was never investigated 20 years ago. On examination, myoclonus is present, he has impaired joint proprioception and vibration, and his pupils are small and do not react to light from a pen-torch. What is the most likely diagnosis?

A. Spinal tuberculosis

B. Creutzfeldt-Jakob disease

C. Tertiary syphilis

D. Frontotemporal dementia

E. Bipolar disorder

29. A 19-year-old male is brought into the A&E after falling and hitting his head on a kerb after a night out. He retained consciousness throughout and can remember the incident. On examination, he has a minor scalp laceration, his GCS is 15/15 with no focal neurological deficit, he is alert, orientated in time, place and person, and he does not complain of any neck stiffness. What is the next management step?

A. CT head scan within 1 hour

B. CT head scan within 8 hours

C. Active neuro-observations, no CT scan indicated

D. X-ray cervical spine

E. MRI brain scan within 24 hours

30. During a ward round, the consultant demonstrates the knee jerk reflex to a group of medical students. What spinal cord level is this reflex testing?

    A. C5-C6

    B. L1-L2

    ● C. L3-L4

    D. L4-L5

    E. S1

31. A patient with multiple sclerosis is suffering with spasticity. Her leg is very tight and has episodes where it 'goes into spasm'. This is causing her considerable distress as she has been falling over at work, and she does not want to draw attention to her diagnosis to her colleagues. What first line medication can be used to reduce her spasticity?

    A. Pyridostigmine

    B. Baclofen

    ● C. Diazepam

    D. Aspirin

    E. Propranolol

32. George, a 32-year-old male, presents to a neurosurgery outpatient clinic. 12 weeks ago, he was playing with his 4-year-old child in the playground and picking her up when he felt a sudden jolt of pain in his back. Since then, the pain has been unbearable and travels down his left-hand side. He says that the back of his leg gets 'hot, cold and now numb'. On examination, he has no pain or tenderness in the back muscles, but has impaired pinprick sensation on the posterolateral aspect of the left leg, with slightly reduced power. What is the most likely diagnosis?

    A. Disc prolapse

    B. Musculoskeletal back pain

    ● C. Cauda equina syndrome

    D. Spinal tumour

    E. Metastatic spinal cord compression

33.   A 20-year-old female is brought into the emergency department, complaining of sudden onset vision loss. On examination, she is visibly shaking and cannot perceive light, but notices and responds to your hand when you raise it into her field of vision. An hour ago, she was in a road traffic accident, where she unfortunately witnessed several fatalities. What is the most likely diagnosis?

A.   Transient ischaemic attack

B.   Giant cell arteritis

C.   Acute stress reaction

D.   Somatisation disorder

E.   Hypertensive emergency

34.   A 32-year-old female with a recent diagnosis of multiple sclerosis (MS) attends a neurology clinic. She has been doing some reading on the internet and would like to know which MS 'clinical pattern' she has. The neurologist tells her that she has the most common pattern of MS. What type does she have?

A.   Primary-progressive

B.   Relapsing-remitting

C.   Secondary-progressive

D.   Progressive-relapsing

E.   Radiologically isolated

35.   Samuel is a 23-year-old student who attends an outpatient first seizure clinic. He was watching TV with his girlfriend when she noticed he was acting strangely, and she took a video which she shows you. You see him stare blankly at the TV before smacking his lips repeatedly and chewing in an irregular fashion. Samuel cannot remember the event, but does recall developing a 'metallic' taste in his mouth 30 minutes beforehand, as well as a strange, funny sensation in his stomach. What location is the seizure he has had?

A.   Frontal lobe

B.   Parietal lobe

C.   Temporal lobe

D.   Occipital lobe

E.   Every lobe (generalised seizure)

36.   A 26-year-old male with cluster headache attends his GP. Over the past 6 weeks, his symptoms have worsened and he now wants to explore medical options to prevent the episodes from occurring. He has no known drug allergies and takes no medication. What should the GP start him on?

A.   Verapamil

B.   Propranolol

C.   Lithium

D.   Lamotrigine

E.   Primidone

37.   What scoring system would be used in an emergency department to assess the possibility of a patient having a stroke and to account for the possibility of stroke mimics?

A.   ABCD2

B.   FAST

C.   NIHSS

D.   ROSIER

E.   GLASGOW

38.   Study the image below. What is the most likely diagnosis?

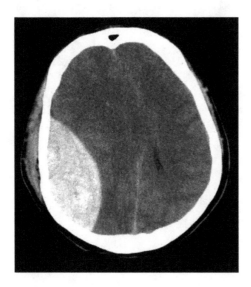

*With permission from Dr Christopher McLeavy, Royal Liverpool and Broadgreen University Hospitals NHS Trust, UK

A.   Acute subdural haematoma

B.   Acute on chronic subdural haematoma

C.   Acute extradural haematoma

D.   Subarachnoid haemorrhage

E.   Chronic subdural haematoma

39.   **Study the image below of a patient who presented with headaches, fever and left-sided weakness, and is a known intravenous drug user. What is the most likely diagnosis?**

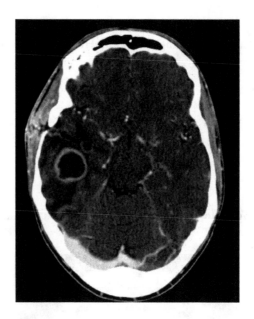

*With permission from Dr Christopher McLeavy, Royal Liverpool and Broadgreen University Hospitals NHS Trust, UK

A.   Glioblastoma

B.   Meningioma

C.   Arteriovenous malformation

D.   Cerebral abscess

E.   Colloid cyst

40.   Doris, an 85-year-old female with a history of heart failure, Type 2 diabetes, and Lewy Body dementia, is recovering from a dynamic hip screw procedure for a fractured neck of femur when she becomes confused and agitated during the ward round the next day. She has been threatening the hospital staff and tried to punch several nurses, and the consultant thinks she has delirium. What is the most appropriate initial treatment?

A.   Lorazepam

B.   L-dopa

 C.   Haloperidol

D.   Chlorpromazine

E.   Morphine sulfate

Practice Paper 3

1. Whilst on a neurology special study module as a final year student doctor, you review a patient with multiple sclerosis in a neurology clinic. She reports that her symptoms get worse in hot weather, and she has occasionally experienced visual loss after going on long bike rides with her partner. What is she describing?

    A. Lhermitte's sign
    B. Hoover's sign
    C. Uhthoff phenomenon
    D. Internuclear ophthalmoplegia
    E. Brudzinski's sign

2. Humayun, a 19-year-old male with epilepsy, starts having a seizure in the waiting room of a GP surgery before a routine vaccination appointment. You arrive and secure his airway, his breathing is constant, and he has now been fitting for 7 minutes. Your GP clinic is in a rural area, so an ambulance will take at least half an hour to arrive. The experienced nurse has attempted intravenous access several times with no success. A finger pinprick glucose measurement is normal. What is the next best management step?

    A. Stabilise airway again, wait for ambulance to arrive
    B. Give 1 mg Intramuscular glucagon
    C. Attempt intravenous access yourself to try and give lorazepam
    D. Commence intramuscular adrenaline
    E. Commence rectal diazepam 10 mg

3. Lucy, a 42-year-old accountant from London, attends her local emergency department with a 3-month history of headache. The headache is worst after she wakes up and when she lies down after a long day at work. Last week, she noticed some double vision, again worst in the morning, and has had 2 episodes of vomiting. Her GP prescribed paracetamol and told her that it was migraine. However, the headache has persisted and is 'getting worse as the days go by'. She is normally fit and well but looks worried. What is the most likely diagnosis?

    A. Benign paroxysmal positional vertigo
    B. Headache due to raised intracranial pressure
    C. Tension headache
    D. Horner's syndrome
    E. Hemiplegic migraine

4.   Tania, a 28-year-old female, has recently been diagnosed with Idiopathic
     intracranial hypertension. What is the most effective first line treatment the
     consultant neurologist will recommend?

     A.   Acetazolamide

     B.   Ventriculoperitoneal shunt

     C.   Endoscopic third ventriculostomy

     D.   Venoplasty

     E.   Weight loss

5.   A 68-year-old male presents to the A&E with sudden onset dizziness and vertigo,
     which happened when he tried to stand up after watching TV 4 hours ago. He
     has a history of hypertension controlled on amlodipine, type 2 diabetes, and atrial
     fibrillation, for which he takes apixaban. An enthusiastic junior doctor attempted
     Hallpike's and Epley's manoeuvre, but this did not resolve the symptoms. This
     episode has never happened before. He reports no hearing loss, tinnitus, headache,
     or weakness, and neurological examination is normal except for severe dizziness,
     which prevents him from standing. What is the most likely diagnosis?

     A.   Posterior circulatory stroke

     B.   Vestibular migraine

     C.   Ménière's disease

     D.   Benign Paroxysmal positional vertigo

     E.   Vestibular neuritis

6.   Fred, a 70-year-old male patient, is in the acute medical ward recovering from a
     large stroke yesterday. This morning on the ward round, the nurses say he was
     agitated last night and not his normal self, and now he is no longer responsive.
     His GCS is 8 on examination, and an emergency CT scan reveals a substantial
     area of infarct occupying 80% of the left middle cerebral artery territory with
     mass effect. What is the best management plan?

     A.   Palliative treatment only

     B.   Nimodipine, urgent stroke team referral

     C.   Intubate and ventilate, urgent stroke team referral

     D.   Intubate and ventilate, urgent neurosurgical referral

     E.   Consider thrombolysis if symptom onset is within time window

7.   After having teaching in the morning and missing the geriatrics ward round, an excited F1 doctor grabs you and demands that you diagnose their patient, who had a stroke last week. On examination, the patient's left eye is fixed, dilated, and unreactive to light. They have significant ptosis and normal power on the left side. While the right eye is normal, there is a dense hemiplegia with MRC grade 0/5 power on the right-hand side of the body. What is the correct diagnosis?

A.   Wallenberg's syndrome (lateral medullary syndrome)

B.   Claude syndrome

C.   Weber syndrome

D.   Gerstmann's syndrome

E.   Millard-Gubler syndrome

8.   You are an F2 doctor on your GP rotation. Your next patient is Rachel, a 72-year-old female, who is accompanied by her husband. He is concerned that for the past year, she has been complaining of seeing 'gnomes' running around the front garden and shouting at them repeatedly. She also seems to 'snap in and out of herself' once every few days, varying from being her normal self to being very forgetful and not remembering to walk their dog, which she had always done previously. On examination, she appears very tired, has a slow gait, and scores 24/30 on the mini mental state examination. What is the most likely diagnosis?

A.   Frontotemporal dementia

B.   Alzheimer's dementia

C.   Lewy body dementia

D.   Depressive pseudodementia

E.   Vascular dementia

9.   You are clerking a young patient in the A&E and you are concerned. For the past week, he has had a fever as well as a seizure before coming to the A&E. His parents had noticed him acting strangely over the last few days. On examination, he appears confused, and you note mild neck stiffness. Based on the most likely diagnosis, what is the next most appropriate management strategy?

A.   Start intravenous ceftriaxone, request senior input

B.   Request an urgent lumbar puncture before giving any treatment

C.   Start intravenous acyclovir, request senior input

D.   Carry out the 'sepsis six'

E.   Start intravenous benzylpenicillin

10. A 5-year-old boy is brought to the paediatric outpatient clinic by his parents after seeing him go through 'weird funny do's'. These episodes last 10 minutes each, occur when they have just put him to bed, and consist of him going stiff and shaking. He cannot remember the episodes but does say that he gets a 'funny feeling', pointing to the right side of his face and tongue after an episode. What is the most likely diagnosis?

A. Absence seizures

B. Benign Rolandic epilepsy

 C. Panayiotopoulos syndrome

D. Infantile spasms (West syndrome)

E. Juvenile myoclonic epilepsy

11. As an F1 on a surgical ward, one of the nurses comes to see you, concerned about one of her patients. Reginald, an 83-year-old male, had an elective cholecystectomy 3 days ago and was recovering well until last night. He was disorientated, shouting at staff and relentlessly climbing out of bed. On the round this morning, he was found asleep but in an awkward position on the bed. His post-op catheter is draining well, has been in for three days, and the fluid in the bag is slightly cloudy. What is the most likely diagnosis?

A. Parkinson medication withdrawal

B. Wernicke's encephalopathy

● C. Lewy body dementia

D. Acute delirium

E. New onset dementia

12. A 22-year-old female patient attends her local GP with altered sensation. On examination, she has normal power, proprioception and vibration of the upper limbs, but diminished sensation to pain and temperature running up the arms. She also has muscle wasting of the small muscles of her hand. Last year, she underwent a foramen magnum decompression for a Chiari malformation. What is the most likely cause of her altered sensation?

A. Side effect of Chiari malformation surgery

B. Thalamic lesion

▲ C. Peripheral neuropathy

D. Subacute combined degeneration of the cord

E. Syringomyelia

13. You are a medical student sitting in a memory clinic as part of a geriatrics rotation, but you notice the next patient is only 28 years old. The consultant explains that he has a past history of severe alcohol misuse and malnutrition, and has now developed the long-term complication of Korsakoff's syndrome. Which of the following is a characteristic feature of the diagnosis?

   A. Reversible with thiamine treatment

   B. Visual hallucinations

   C. Fluctuating consciousness level

   D. Psychotic delusions

   E. Anterograde amnesia

14. Arish, a 58-year-old male, presents to his GP with 'stinging' leg pain. The pain starts at the side of his thigh and travels down quickly to his knee, and he also complains of 'a funny tingling feeling' when the pain comes on. His past medical history includes a TIA aged 48 and poorly controlled type 2 diabetes, and his latest HbA1c is 88 (normal range ≤48) despite being on insulin. He rarely exercises, and his body mass index is 35. What is the most likely diagnosis?

   A. Peripheral neuropathy due to diabetes

   B. Greater trochanteric pain syndrome (trochanteric bursitis)

   C. Meralgia paraesthesia

   D. Diabetic amyotrophy

   E. Polymyositis

15. Chris, a 21-year-old medical student, comes to your GP being very anxious and concerned about 'my tremor'. He has been learning about Parkinson's disease as part of his introduction to neurology block and is worried that he might have it. His grandfather had Parkinson's diagnosed at age 70, but there is no other family history. Apart from irritable bowel syndrome, he is normally fit and well and takes no medications. He says thinking and worrying about the tremor makes it worse, but he does notice an improvement when he goes on nights out for medic's rugby social events and has a few drinks. On examination, he has a tremor that worsens when he tries to touch your finger, which resolves at rest. What is the most likely diagnosis?

   A. Benign essential tremor

   B. Rubral (Holmes) tremor

   C. Familial early onset Parkinson's disease

   D. Medication induced tremor

   E. Anxiety

16. After successfully diagnosing Chris, what treatment is most appropriate to commence?

A. Levodopa

B. Amitriptyline

C. Propranolol

D. Dopamine receptor agonists (e.g., ropinirole)

E. Daily low dose alcohol

17. Which of the following may cause lower motor neuron signs on examination?

A. Stroke

B. Brain tumours

C. Multiple sclerosis

D. Bulbar palsy

E. Pseudobulbar palsy

18. As an F2 doctor, you are working in a paediatrics ward and you see a 3-year-old boy with intractable epilepsy. Extensive investigations have been ordered including an EEG, but his parents say the cause has not been found. They also mention that he has been globally behind with his development from a young age. On examination, you notice a facial rash as well as a discrete scaly rash across his lower back. What is the most likely cause of his epilepsy?

A. Neurofibromatosis

B. Ohtahara syndrome

C. Sturge-Weber syndrome

D. Intracranial tumour

E. Tuberous sclerosis

19. You have just observed a brain tumour removal in an adult patient in the neurosurgical theatre. The next day, the consultant reads to you the pathology report which states, 'The tumour shows marked brain invasion and crosses the corpus callosum on imaging, with areas of extreme vascularity and necrosis, and is the most aggressive primary brain tumour'. What was the tumour type?

A. Meningioma

B. Haemangioblastoma

C. Anaplastic astrocytoma

D. Cavernoma

E. Glioblastoma

20.   Which of the following could be a cause of visual loss noted as 'bitemporal hemianopia'?

   A.   Pituitary adenoma

   B.   Multiple sclerosis

   ▲   C.   Optic nerve glioma

   D.   Stroke

   E.   Occipital cortex tumour

21.   You are on placement in the intensive care unit, when the consultant intensivist asks you to diagnose a long-term patient who was admitted after a severe head injury sustained in a skiing accident. She tells you that the patient still has sleep-wake cycles, opens their eyes but cannot make any purposeful movements, and cannot communicate by any means. What is the most likely diagnosis?

   A.   Coma

   B.   Brainstem death

   ▲   C.   Persistent vegetative state

   D.   Locked in syndrome

   E.   Minimally conscious state

22.   You are on a weekend run when you see a large road traffic accident, and you go over and offer to help. You find a young male patient with severe bleeding from a scalp wound. He opens his eyes to pain, makes vague groaning noises, and on applying a pain stimulus, his right arm extends away from the pain site. What is the most appropriate next management step?

   A.   Stabilise airway, check blood glucose

   B.   Stabilise airway, consider intubation and ventilation when possible

   ●   C.   Needle cricothyrotomy

   D.   Surgical cricothyrotomy

   E.   Nasopharyngeal tube

23.   A patient is diagnosed with malignant spinal cord compression. What vertebrae is most likely to be affected?

   A.   Cervical

   B.   Thoracic

   ■   C.   Lumbar

   D.   Sacral

   E.   None of the above

24.   Amelia, a 43-year-old English teacher, is admitted to the A&E after suffering a
        seizure. She had suffered from a 'horrendous headache' for 5 minutes immediately
        prior to the seizure. A CT head scan shows a large volume of intracerebral
        haemorrhage, but no evidence of blood in the subarachnoid space. A magnetic
        resonance angiography scan reveals a tortuous collection of blood vessels within
        the haemorrhage with a central nidus, and is labelled a 'Spetzler-Martin grade 2'.
        What is the diagnosis?

        A.   Cavernoma

        B.   Subarachnoid haemorrhage

 C.   Arachnoid cyst rupture

        D.   Arteriovenous malformation

        E.   Lobar haemorrhage

25.   You are a newly qualified doctor on a neurosurgical ward, and on the ward round
        you see a patient who suffered a subarachnoid haemorrhage. The registrar
        asks you to order bloods to look for a specific complication of the haemorrhage
        before running off to theatre without his bleep. What blood test should you
        order?

        A.   Haemoglobin levels

 B.   Urea and electrolytes

        C.   ESR and CRP

        D.   Autoimmune screen

        E.   Liver function tests

26.   You are investigating a patient with a suspected anterior communicating artery
        aneurysm. What is the best investigation to assist in making the diagnosis?

        A.   Carotid doppler

        B.   MRI brain scan

        C.   CT angiography

        D.   CT head scan

        E.   Cranial ultrasound scan

27.   Lisa, a 21-year-old female, attends her GP with a persistent headache for the past
        6 months. It is located near the back of her head in the occipital region and is
        worse when she coughs or lies flat. She has a history of myelomeningocele (spina
        bifida), but is otherwise well. An outpatient MRI scan shows no masses or lesions,
        but does demonstrate a displaced lower cerebellum with mild compression of the
        foramen magnum. What is the most likely diagnosis?

        A.   Chiari malformation

        B.   Brain tumour

        C.   Idiopathic intracranial hypertension

        D.   Benign occipital headache

        E.   Atlantoaxial subluxation

28.   Your next patient in the GP surgery is Graham, an 81-year-old male. His wife
        strongly believes he has dementia as he has been forgetting to turn the hobs off
        the stove or walk the family golden retriever, and he keeps getting lost in familiar
        streets. Graham denies this and says his wife is 'out to get him'. He does not seem
        concerned and would rather talk about his recent incontinence issues — he has
        had to wear adult nappies for the last year — and says that 'it can't be a part of
        getting older'. As they leave, you note that he has a slow gait and appears clumsy
        on his feet. What is the most likely diagnosis?

        A.   Alzheimer's disease

        B.   Benign prostatic hyperplasia

        C.   Frontotemporal dementia

        D.   Mild cognitive impairment

        E.   Normal pressure hydrocephalus

29.   A patient with newly diagnosed Parkinson's disease is started on ropinirole (a
        dopamine agonist) by his neurologist. What potential side effect should they be
        warned about most?

        A.   Postural hypotension

        B.   Gambling disorders and hypersexuality

        C.   Diarrhoea

        D.   Taste disturbance

        E.   Reduced seizure threshold

30.   A 45-year-old female attends the emergency department after being sent by her GP. Over the past few days, her multiple sclerosis symptoms have been worsening, she has had paraesthesia affecting the left leg, and her vision is blurred. On examination, her visual acuity is 6/6 in the right eye and 6/60 in the left eye. Apart from paraesthesia, her motor examination is normal with normal power. What is the most appropriate management?

     A.   Acetazolamide

     B.   Natalizumab

     C.   Alemtuzumab

     D.   Pulsed methylprednisolone

     E.   Glatiramer acetate

31.   A 21-year-old male is under investigation for a series of suspicious 'episodes'. They last 3–5 minutes and involve his right arm and leg spontaneously twitching. He can remember the episodes and does not lose consciousness when experiencing them. What is the diagnosis?

     A.   Focal aware seizure

     B.   Complex partial seizure

     C.   Generalised tonic-clonic seizure

     D.   Absence seizure

     E.   Non-epileptic attack (psychogenic seizure)

32.   A 28-year-old female attends the GP with severe headaches. On taking a detailed history, she describes them as starting in her early teens, and she found that taking paracetamol or ibuprofen would 'take the edge off'. She has no auras, visual disturbances, weakness, or numbness. She currently takes paracetamol, ibuprofen, and amitriptyline every day for these headaches, and has been following this regime for the last 6 months. She is otherwise fit and well. Given the likely diagnosis, what is the best management plan for her?

     A.   Continue regular medications, add propranolol

     B.   Increase paracetamol dose, discontinue other medications

     C.   Slowly reduce doses of all medications with a plan to discontinue all of them

     D.   Stop all medications, then start topiramate

     E.   Add sodium valproate, continue all other medications

33.   As a final year medical student, you and your F1 doctor are called to attend to a patient who suffered a seizure 5 minutes ago. The seizure has terminated, and they are now rousable and slowly recovering. The attending consultant asks the F1 to order a blood test that may help to differentiate between a seizure and a psychogenic seizure. Which blood test should the F1 request?

A.   Lactate

B.   Prolactin

C.   Mast cell tryptase

D.   Ferritin

E.   Urea and electrolytes

34.   A patient attends a specialist nurse follow up appointment after suffering a stroke 2 weeks ago. Her partner tells the nurse that she presented with left-sided weakness that affected her leg, with her arm relatively spared, sudden urinary incontinence, and personality change. Which artery has been affected by the stroke?

A.   Anterior communicating artery

B.   Anterior cerebral artery

C.   Middle cerebral artery

D.   Posterior inferior cerebellar artery

E.   Posterior cerebral artery

35.   Whilst on a psychiatry placement, you encounter a patient who has a long-standing history of alcohol misuse. They presented originally with Wernicke's encephalopathy, but Korsakoff's syndrome has unfortunately developed as a result. Which vitamin is deficient to cause both of these conditions?

A.   Thiamine (vitamin B1)

B.   Niacin (vitamin B3)

C.   Vitamin B6

D.   Vitamin C

E.   Vitamin B12

36.   A 62-year-old male patient attends the GP for a review after having a stroke whilst on holiday in Tenerife 2 weeks ago. The patient was managed conservatively and his left-sided weakness has since improved. The patient mentions that the doctors in Tenerife told him to ask his GP to prescribe long-term medication to prevent further strokes. His inpatient hospital admission form notes that he suffered a severe allergic reaction to Clopidogrel when he was started on it by the hospital team. What medication would you commence him on?

A.   Clopidogrel 75 mg OD

B.   Aspirin 300 mg for 2 weeks, then 75 mg

C.   Aspirin 75 mg and modified release dipyridamole

D.   Do not commence any medication until an ABCD2 score has been calculated

E.   Apixaban 5 mg

37.   A patient presents with unique clinical features and signs of finger agnosia, agraphia, and acalculia, as well as confusion between the right- and left-hand side. What is the name for this syndrome?

A.   Weber syndrome

B.   Gerstmann's syndrome

C.   Wallenberg syndrome

D.   Parinaud syndrome

E.   Claude syndrome

38.   A 22-year-old male university student attends the emergency department looking very unwell. For the past 3 days, he has been generally unwell, has not been eating, and has a severe headache. His flatmates have noticed that he has been in his room with the lights off for the past few days. On examination, he is barely rousable, his neck is held in position, and he grabs his neck in pain when extending a flexed knee at the hip. What is the most likely diagnosis?

A.   Encephalitis

B.   Carbon monoxide poisoning

C.   Meningitis

D.   Guillain-Barré syndrome

E.   Subdural haematoma

39.   A patient attends the emergency department and receives the CT head scan shown below:

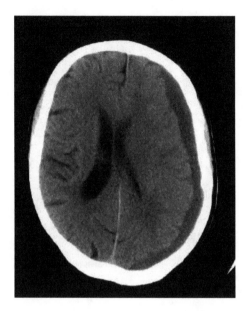

What is the most likely diagnosis?

A. Acute extradural haematoma

B. Hydrocephalus

C. Chronic subdural haematoma

D. Acute on chronic subdural haematoma

E. Hydrocephalus

40.   A patient attends the emergency department with reduced consciousness level and receives the CT head scan shown below:

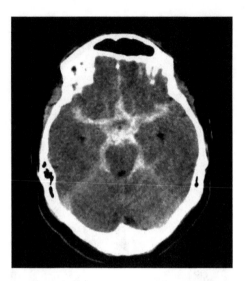

What is the most likely diagnosis?

A.   Cerebral contusion

B.   Skull fracture

C.   Normal scan with contrast

D.   Hydrocephalus

E.   Subarachnoid haemorrhage

Practice Paper 4

1. A 23-year-old male patient presents to the GP with a new onset headache for the past two days. It is worse when he stands up from a sitting or lying position, and he has been feeling quite drained since the headache started. The headache improves when bending down and lying flat, and he has no photophobia or visual changes. He is normally fit and well, and he underwent a lumbar puncture 4 days ago when he was admitted to hospital with a meningitis scare, which turned out negative. What is the most likely diagnosis?

    A. Headache due to raised intracranial pressure

    B. Cluster headache

     C. Post-coital headache

    D. Paroxysmal hemicrania

    E. Low pressure headache

2. A 43-year-old male is currently a long-term patient in the intensive care unit after suffering respiratory failure as a complication of Guillain-Barré syndrome. You are asked to review his neurological function. On examination, you note that he does not have any voluntary movement, but has sleep wake cycles and can still communicate using eye blinking movements. What is the diagnosis?

    A. Brainstem death

    B. Minimally conscious state

    ● C. Persistent vegetative state

    D. Coma

    E. Locked in syndrome

3. A 53-year-old female smoker attends the GP clinic with back pain. For the past 12 weeks she has had pain mostly on her left-hand side, which travels down her left leg. She also describes developing a numb feeling on the dorsum of her foot during this time. There was no trigger and she did not have any recent falls. She was started on NSAIDs and paracetamol, but this has not helped her symptoms. She works as a primary school teacher. The GP suspects a diagnosis of disc herniation. What is the best investigation to diagnose this?

    A. Straight leg raise test

    B. Outpatient MRI lumbosacral spine

    ● C. CT spine scan

    D. PET-CT scan

    E. Lumbar puncture

4. An 86-year-old male is admitted to the hospital after falling when climbing a ladder to tend to his shrubbery. He remembers the fall, and his wife witnessed him hitting his head on the grass. He did not lose consciousness, is alert but complains of significant pain, and is bruised on his left cheek. He is a retired army sergeant and scores 28/30 on the MMSE. He states that he feels okay and would like to go home. What is the next appropriate management step?

    A. Discharge him home

    B. CT head scan within 1 hour

    C. CT head scan within 8 hours

    D. Neuro-observations for next 24 hrs, no scan needed

    E. Send him home and arrange for outpatient MRI

5. You are asked to examine the cranial nerves of a patient in the neurology clinic. On examination, when asking the patient to look to the left, the right eye moves but the left eye remains stationary. When asked to move to the right, the left eye and right eye both move to the right. All other components of the examination are normal and the pupil size is regular. What is the most likely diagnosis?

    A. Right oculomotor nerve palsy

    B. Left oculomotor nerve palsy

    C. Right abducens nerve palsy

    D. Left abducens nerve palsy

    E. Right trochlear nerve palsy

6. A 54-year-old female presents to your GP clinic complaining of hearing loss. This has been troubling her for the last 3 months, but her husband thinks 'she is just getting old'. She has no other symptoms. On examination, you note that Rinne's test is louder when placed in front of the ear for the right-hand side and is not heard on the left-hand side. Weber's test is heard loudest in the right ear. An audiogram confirms the hearing loss pattern observed on examination. What is the next best investigation to perform, given the likely diagnosis?

    A. Repeat audiogram in 2 months

    B. ENT appointment for hearing aid fitting

    C. Hallpike and Epley manoeuvres

    D. Urgent CT head scan

    E. Urgent MRI of the cerebellopontine angle

7. While in a fifth year OSCE, you are asked to perform a sensory examination of the lower limb. After you finish the examination, the examiner asks you what dermatome is represented by the medial side of the leg. What answer should you give her?

   A. L2

   B. L3

   C. L4

   D. L5

   E. S1

8. A 63-year-old male attends a TIA rapid access clinic after experiencing a transient episode of left arm weakness. This episode started whilst watching a football game and resolved 15 minutes later. He did not have speech disturbances or any other symptoms. His regular medications are listed as atorvastatin for high cholesterol and amlodipine for hypertension. He does not have diabetes. What is his ABCD^2 score?

   A. 1

   B. 2

   C. 3

   D. 4

   E. 5

9. A 27-year-old male attends the emergency department in a dishevelled state. His address is listed as a local hostel in the city centre. His friend mentions that he has been confused and agitated for the past 2 days, and he had been complaining of a headache. He has a history of latent tuberculosis with poor compliance with treatment medications. On examination, you note needle track marks in his antecubital fossae, he appears unkempt, and his temperature is 38.9°C, with all other observations normal. A CT head scan reveals a well-circumscribed and defined ring-enhancing lesion in the left frontal lobe, with no mass effect or surrounding oedema. What is the most likely diagnosis?

   A. Cerebral abscess

   B. Glioblastoma

   C. Progressive multifocal leukoencephalopathy

   D. Wernicke's encephalopathy

   E. Intracerebral haemorrhage

10. A 21-year-old male patient attends the emergency department with a headache. He has had repeated episodes of cluster headache in the past 3 months, and they have now gotten worse to the point of being unbearable today. What is the most appropriate management of his headache?

    A. Botulinum toxin injections

    B. Buccal midazolam

    C. High flow oxygen and sumatriptan

    D. Propranolol and paracetamol

    E. Verapamil stat dose

11. A 32-year-old male who is normally fit and well attends the out-of-hours urgent care centre with left-sided weakness. Apart from a rough day with the kids yesterday where he was turning his head around a lot while chasing them, he has no triggers. On examination, all of his observations are normal including heart rate and blood pressure. He has considerable right-sided weakness (MRC grade 2) in the upper and lower limbs. An MRI head scan arranged the next day shows an area of infarction in the middle cerebral artery territory. What is the most likely cause of his stroke?

    A. Homocystinuria

    B. Carotid dissection

    C. CADASIL

    D. Tertiary syphilis

    E. Multiple sclerosis

12. As a fourth year medical student, you are asked to interpret a lumbar puncture report of Doris, a 68-year-old female, who has presented with a vague history of fever, headache, and neurological decline.

Opening pressure (cmH$_2$O): Raised

White cell count: 15.9 (Raised), 50% Neutrophils

Glucose: 1.2 (Low)

Gram stain: Gram-positive rod identified

India ink stain: Negative

Colour: Turbid

What is the most likely causative organism?

A. Neisseria meningitidis

B. E. coli

 C. Listeria monocytogenes

D. Viral

E. Mycoplasma tuberculosis

13. A 65-year-old female attends a GP complaining of facial weakness. This started when she woke up this morning to find that the left side of her face had 'drooped over' and she thought she was having a stroke. However, she had no weakness and her speech was fine, so she decided to go to the GP instead. On examination, she has no weakness, but the left-hand side of her face is 'dropping down'. She cannot close her left eye and there is loss of wrinkles on the left-hand side of her forehead. What is the most likely diagnosis?

A. Lacunar stroke

B. Ramsay Hunt syndrome

C. Motor neurone disease

D. Bell's palsy

E. Trigeminal neuralgia

14. You are watching a video during a clinical skills session showing different gaits. The next patient is middle aged and, on walking, appears to swing their affected legs around and flexes their leg before placing it on the ground. What kind of gait does this patient have?

A. Trendelenburg gait

B. Circumduction

C. Waddling gait

D. Spastic gait

E. Neuropathic gait

15.   A 2-day-old neonate is referred to the paediatric neurosurgery team as the local
       women's hospital had concerns. He is feeding poorly and has been drowsy since
       birth with a weak, high pitched cry. The neonate was delivered by emergency
       C-section at 28 weeks due to signs of fetal compromise. On examination, you
       note an enlarged head circumference, the veins around his scalp appear grossly
       dilated, and his eyes remain fixed in a downward position. What is the most likely
       diagnosis?

       A.   Anencephaly
       B.   Myelomeningocele
 C.   Encephalocele
       D.   Cerebral palsy
       E.   Hydrocephalus

16.   A 19-year-old female university student attends her university GP complaining
       of becoming increasingly clumsy over the past few months. She is normally fit
       and well, exercises regularly, and has had a strict vegan diet from the age of 15.
       On examination, she has an unsteady gait, lower limb weakness, and impaired
       awareness to proprioception, and when a tuning fork is placed on her toe, she
       cannot feel it. Her knee reflexes are absent, but her ankle jerks are brisk. What is
       the most likely diagnosis?

       A.   Drug-induced peripheral neuropathy
       B.   Tabes dorsalis
●   C.   Inherited motor neurone disease
       D.   Subacute combined degeneration of the cord
       E.   Diabetic neuropathy

17.   You are on the ward as a medical student, and you take a history of a 42-year-old
       female who attended the A&E for left-sided weakness. This came on suddenly
       over an hour or so, and she also describes a 'tingling' feeling on the left-hand side
       as well as a dull, persistent headache that she has had for some time. On
       examination, she has dense hemiparesis with MRC grade 2/5 power on the left
       upper and lower limbs. Sensation, cranial nerves, and speech are all normal.
       A CT head scan obtained acutely was negative, and an MRI brain scan taken an
       hour ago is normal. What is the most likely diagnosis?

       A.   Acute stroke
       B.   Subarachnoid haemorrhage
■   C.   Conversion disorder
       D.   Multiple sclerosis
       E.   Hemiplegic migraine

18. A consultant is quizzing you on rare headache types. She describes a headache that feels like an 'icepick' on the skin and has a characteristic response to the medication indomethacin. What type of headache is she describing?

    A. Paroxysmal hemicrania
    B. Cluster headache
    C. SUNCT
    D. Atypical migraine
    E. Thunderclap headache

19. You are on the ward when a nurse asks for your help. A 48-year-old male has presented to the A&E with severe vertigo. He has a known diagnosis of benign paroxysmal positional vertigo and says this is similar. Which manoeuvre may help treat this patient?

    A. Epley
    B. Dix-Hallpike
    C. Romberg
    D. Smith
    E. Jacobsen's

20. A 2-year-old girl is brought into the GP surgery by her mother. She was delivered through an emergency C-section following an antepartum haemorrhage and is globally behind on her milestones. On examination, she has a spastic gait, with weakness of both legs which have increased tone. Which subtype of cerebral palsy does the patient have?

    A. Spastic diplegic
    B. Ataxic
    C. Dyskinetic cerebral palsy
    D. Quadriplegic cerebral palsy

21. You are asked to examine the pupils of a patient. The patient's pupils do not react to light, but when you perform the 'swinging light' test, her pupils dilate. Where is the lesion or cause of her pupil abnormality?

    A. Optic chiasm
    B. Optic radiation
    C. Optic nerve
    D. Paramedian pontine reticular formation
    E. Occipital cortex

22.   A 22-year-old male attends his local GP with his mother. She says he has not been
        himself for the last few months, being more forgetful and irritable than usual. He
        plays for the university's rugby team and admits to taking a few hard hits during
        the season. What is the most likely diagnosis?

        A.   No pathology
        B.   Post-concussion syndrome
        C.   Early onset dementia
        D.   Bipolar disorder
        E.   Somatisation disorder

23.   Karen, a 53-year-old female, attends the GP complaining of 'tingling in her hands'.
        She describes numbness in her left hand with a 'dull' feeling. There is no associated
        weakness, although it has been going on for 6 months and is now disrupting her
        work as an NHS typist. She has a past history of hypothyroidism for which she
        takes thyroxine, but is otherwise well. On examination, there is no hand muscle
        wasting, but flexing her hand for thirty seconds produces the same 'dull' feeling.
        What is the most likely diagnosis?

        A.   Ulnar nerve palsy
        B.   Radial nerve palsy
        C.   Median nerve palsy
        D.   Syringomyelia
        E.   Diabetic neuropathy

24.   A patient who has been taking long-term antipsychotics for paranoid schizophrenia
        is diagnosed with tardive dyskinesia. Which medication is essential to avoid in
        this case?

        A.   Procyclidine
        B.   Domperidone
        C.   Propranolol
        D.   Ezetimibe
        E.   Ciprofloxacin

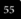

25.   You are working as a junior doctor in a medical ward. You are called to see a patient whose consciousness level has rapidly declined over the last four hours. She presented 2 days ago with confusion and was found to have a urinary tract infection, and her sodium was 120 mmol/l. The on-call SHO set up rehydration with 1L of NaCl 0.9% and her sodium levels increased to 130 mmol/l over the next 12 hours. Her other observations were normal up until this point. What is the most likely diagnosis?

A. Sepsis

B. Worsening of UTI

C. Spontaneous subarachnoid haemorrhage

D. Progressive multifocal leukoencephalopathy

E. Central pontine myelinolysis

26.   A patient presents to the emergency department with sudden onset facial weakness after waking up this morning. You also notice a strange, bumpy vesicular rash on her ear, and she has reported reduced hearing during this time. What is the most likely diagnosis?

A. Bell's palsy

B. Ramsay Hunt syndrome

C. Gorlin syndrome

D. Acute stroke

E. Neuromyelitis optica

27.   You are the junior doctor in the A&E when a 32-year-old male presents with a 4-hour history of sudden onset back pain, leg weakness, and urinary retention. The neurological examination reveals MRC grade 4/5 power in both legs, and he cannot feel a pinprick sensation in the peri-anal area. An urgent MRI confirms that the cauda equina is being compressed. His performance status is zero. What is the best management of this patient?

A. Lie facing up before commencing any management

B. Dexamethasone 4mg

C. Intravenous alteplase

D. Urgent neurosurgical decompression

E. Oncology referral

28.   A 72-year-old patient with a history of 3 cardiac stents and previous coronary artery bypass graft operation presents with acute onset vertigo and double vision. On examination you note loss of facial sensation to pinprick and temperature on the left side of the face, as well as loss of pain and temperature on the right-hand side of the body. What artery territory has been affected?

   A.   Right middle cerebral artery

   B.   Right anterior cerebral artery

▲ C.   Left middle cerebral artery

   D.   Left medial medullary

   E.   Left lateral medullary

29.   A 76-year-old female attends the GP 'feeling a bit funny' after she spent the day fixing a lightbulb with her head up, describing generalised weakness ever since. On examination you note that she has MRC grade 3/5 power in the arms and 5/5 in both legs, and her speech is completely normal. What is the most likely diagnosis?

   A.   Anterior cord syndrome

   B.   Central cord syndrome

■ C.   Syringomyelia

   D.   Brown Sequard syndrome

   E.   Spinal shock

30.   A patient is being investigated for suspected myaesthenia gravis. So far, they have had no investigations besides routine bloods, which have all come back normal. What would be the best investigation to perform next?

   A.   Electromyography

   B.   CT thorax

■ C.   Edrophonium (tensilon) test

   D.   MRI head scan

   E.   Lumbar puncture

31.   A 24-year-old male presents to the A&E with generalised weakness and respiratory distress. He is normally fit and well with no past medical history, but he does recall having an episode of bad diarrhoea two weeks ago. The weakness started in his upper limbs before moving downwards. On examination, he has an unsteady gait, MRC grade 2/5 power throughout with reduced tendon reflexes, and limited eye movement globally. What is the most likely diagnosis?

   A.   First onset multiple sclerosis

   B.   Guillain-Barré syndrome

   C.   Subacute sclerosing panencephalitis

   D.   Transverse myelitis

   E.   Miller-Fischer syndrome

32.   A 63-year-old male with treatment refractory Parkinson's disease attends the neurology outpatient clinic and you take a medication history. He describes how he was diagnosed 15 years ago and was started on levodopa followed by ropinirole (dopamine agonist), before moving on to other complex treatment regimens as his treatment progressed. Lately, his main problem has been periods where he is 'frozen', but he also tells you that this has reduced after starting a new medication. The consultant informs you that this is a last resort medication and it is a rapidly acting dopamine agonist. What medication has he been taking?

   A.   No medication — he has had deep brain stimulation

   B.   Intrajejunal duodopa

   C.   Selegeline

   D.   Apomorphine

   E.   Cabergoline

33.   You are taking a history from a patient with epilepsy, and he describes his usual seizure pattern as starting with a metallic taste in his mouth and a 'funny feeling' in his stomach, following which he cannot remember what he does. His partner states that he walks around the room seemingly without purpose, moving his head in different directions, and smacking his lips repeatedly. What type of seizure does he have?

   A.   Focal-impaired awareness

   B.   Focal-aware

   C.   Generalised tonic-clonic

   D.   Generalised absence

   E.   Complex partial

34.   On a ward round, a stroke patient is recovering after undergoing thrombolysis yesterday for a left PACS. The patient recovered complete functioning after thrombolysis and is due to be discharged today. The nurse comes over to inform you that the consultant has prescribed antiplatelet therapy, but has not stated when the patient should start taking it. How long after thrombolysis should you wait before starting antiplatelet therapy?

A.   Give immediately

B.   Wait 24 hours

C.   Wait one week

D.   Wait two weeks

E.   One month

35.   You observe a lumbar puncture on a 19-year-old female with suspected meningitis. The cerebrospinal fluid results are shown below:

Opening pressure (cmH$_2$O): 40 (normal range 5–20)

Appearance: Turbid

Protein (g/L): 2 (normal range 0.18–0.45)

WCC: 2000, 90% polymorpho nucleocytes

Lymphocytes: Normal

Glucose: 1.2 (normal range 2.5–3.5)

Gram stain: Gram-negative cocci

Which of the following organisms is the cause of her meningitis?

A.   Bacterial

B.   Viral

C.   mycobacterium TB

D.   Cryptococcal

E.   Listeria

36.   A 43-year-old male patient presents with fever, confusion, and headaches. He has
       a past history of tuberculosis, oesophageal candidiasis, and cytomegalovirus
       infection. Examination reveals that he is confused, and a friend says he has been
       like this for the last week. A CT head scan reveals a cystic lesion in the parietal
       lobe with prominent intracerebral calcifications. Which of the following is the
       most likely diagnosis?

       A.   Cerebral abscess

       B.   Toxoplasmosis

   ▲   C.   Progressive multifocal leukoencephalopathy

       D.   CNS lymphoma

       E.   Cryptococcal meningitis

37.   A 1-day-old neonate is transferred to the paediatric neurosurgery team and
       undergoes an operation the same day. Her antenatal notes include an abnormality
       that was picked up at a 20-week anomaly scan, and on delivery the patient had
       an open defect in the lumbar region with no covering sac, with elements of the
       spinal cord exposed. What condition did she have immediate surgery for?

       A.   Encephalocele

       B.   Meningocele

   ▲   C.   Myelomeningocele

       D.   Anencephaly

       E.   Spina bifida occulta

38.   A patient presents with weakness on the left side of the face, but strangely has
       weakness of the upper and lower limbs on the right side of their body, and their
       left-hand side is neurologically intact. Where is the lesion most likely to be located?

       A.   Cerebrum

       B.   Brainstem

   ■   C.   Spinal cord

       D.   Ventricles

       E.   Cavernous sinus

39.   A 5-year-old boy is brought into the paediatric A&E department after a 4-week
        history of progressive headache and vomiting. The attending paediatric registrar
        notes papilledema on examination. The emergency CT head scan taken 30 minutes
        after admission is shown below:

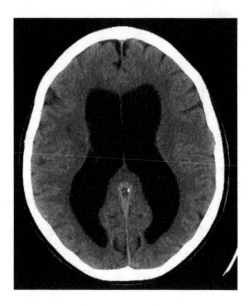

Based on the imaging, what is the most likely diagnosis?

A. Pneumocephalus

B. Hydrocephalus

C. Malignant MCA syndrome

D. Colloid cyst

E. Frontal space-occupying lesion

40.   You take a history from a 74-year-old female, who is currently an inpatient in the long-term neurological rehabilitation ward. After the history, you assess one of her scans on a ward computer. A CT head scan obtained 6 months ago is shown below:

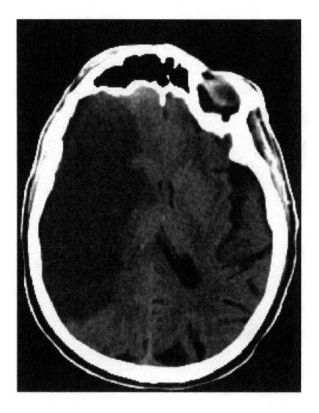

Based on the imaging, why is she in the neuro-rehab ward?

A.   CT head scan not conclusive

B.   Space-occupying lesion with prominent oedema

C.   Vascular dementia

D.   Massive infarction

E.   Recovering from a craniectomy operation

Practice Paper 5

1. A 31-year-old female patient attends the accident and emergency department with her friends, who believe she is having a stroke as her left-hand side has gone completely limp. She has a past history of focal seizures, with her last seizure being 16 hours ago. On examination, she has a dense left-sided monoplegia affecting the lower limb, with MRC grade 0 power. She also appears groggy, but is orientated in time and person and her speech is normal. What is the most likely diagnosis?

    A. Acute stroke
    B. Hemiplegic migraine
    ▲   C. Todd's paresis
    D. Sepsis
    E. Post-syncopal paralysis

2. A 65-year-old male, who is being treated conservatively for stage four small cell lung cancer, presents with a 2-week history of 'weakness'. On examination, he has generalised weakness, but this improves remarkably after repetitive testing. What is the best management option for this patient?

    A. 3, 4 dipyridylamine
    B. Surgery and chemotherapy for small cell cancer
    ■   C. Prednisolone
    D. MRI thorax to look for thymoma
    E. Pyridostigmine

3. A 52-year-old male presents with an episode of 'passing out'. Before the episode, he complained of dizziness and has experienced intermittent palpitations over the previous 6 weeks, as well as 'tightness' of the chest that is worse when walking up the hill to his house. He had no urinary or bowel incontinence afterwards, and recovered consciousness quickly after the episode. What is the likely cause of the patient's syncope?

    A. Vasovagal syncope
    B. Carotid sinus syncope
    ●   C. Seizure
    D. Postural hypotension
    E. Cardiac arrythmia

4.   A patient in clinic has the classical triad of ptosis, miosis, and facial anhidrosis, and you diagnose Horner's syndrome to the delight of your registrar. To your horror, she asks you a follow up question: Which of the following is not a cause of Horner's syndrome?

A.   Multiple sclerosis

B.   Myaesthenia gravis

▲   C.   Lung cancer

D.   Carotid dissection

E.   Cavernous sinus thrombosis

5.   A 62-year-old male has recently been diagnosed with mild dementia and is commenced on Donepezil after counselling. What characteristic side effect may he suffer from?

A.   Dizziness

B.   Headache

■   C.   Diarrhoea

D.   Constipation

E.   Urinary incontinence

6.   A 33-year-old afro-Caribbean female presents with symptoms characteristic of optic neuritis, with symptoms affecting both eyes, and an acute episode of leg weakness that resolved spontaneously. A lumbar puncture, however, is negative for oligoclonal bands but positive for anti-aquaporin antibodies. An MRI scan reveals high-signal periventricular lesions. Which of the following is the most likely diagnosis for this young woman?

A.   Multiple sclerosis

B.   Transverse myelitis

▲   C.   Neuromyelitis optica

D.   Idiopathic intracranial hypertension (IIH)

E.   Complex migraine

7.   A patient presents with speech difficulty. On examination, they can understand, comprehend, and repeat with normal verbal fluency what you say. However, their speech is markedly slurred, almost impeding interpretation. What best describes this defect?

A.   Dysarthria

B.   Dysphasia

C.   Dysmetria

D.   Dysgeusia

E.   Dysphonia

8.   A patient presents with a 6-week history of weakness. On further questioning, she states that she feels weak 'all over' and nothing in particular brought it on. On examination, you find hip flexion and extension to be severely weak, with slightly reduced ankle power. There are no visible scars or rashes. What is the most likely diagnosis?

A.   Polymyositis

B.   Myositis

C.   Guillain-Barré syndrome

D.   Motor neurone disease

E.   Progressive supranuclear palsy

9.   A 43-year-old female attends an outpatient oncology appointment. Her main complaint is that she has issues with her legs, reporting a tingling sensation with occasional numbness. On examination, she has reduced sensation to all modalities in a 'glove and stocking' distribution. Last month, she completed a cycle of prolonged chemotherapy for breast cancer. Which of the following drugs could be a cause of her symptoms?

A.   Doxorubicin

B.   Cisplatin

C.   Vincristine

D.   Docetaxel

E.   Bevacizumab

10.   You are asked to examine a hospital day case patient with multiple sclerosis who has 'unusual' eye signs before his routine clinic appointment. On examination, his pupils are normal and react to light, and his fundoscopy and visual fields are normal. However, when he is asked to look to the left, his right eye does not move, and you notice nystagmus of his left eye. Where is the most likely location of the pathology that is causing this condition?

A.   Spinal cord

B.   Optic nerve

C.   Optic tract

D.   Optic radiation

E.   Medial longitudinal fasciculus

11.   A 45-year-old male presents to his GP with a 6-week history of restlessness. He describes the urge to move his limbs constantly and finds it almost impossible to keep them stationary — this is involuntary and out of his control. He has a past history of paranoid schizophrenia since the age of 40 and is currently on active treatment for this condition. What is the most appropriate treatment for his restlessness?

A.   Procyclidine

B.   Donepezil

C.   Galantamine

D.   Apomorphine

E.   Haloperidol

12.   While on a ward round in a small district hospital, you see a 20-year-old female university student who, for the past two weeks, has been admitted with 'unexplained clumsiness and left leg weakness'. She is normally fit and well, has been studying at a prestigious local university, and has her geography final year exams coming up. The neurology consultant comes to see her. On examination, she has MRC grade 5 power in both the upper and lower limbs, and her tone, reflexes, and sensory examination are all normal. When asked to walk, she takes odd, circumducted gaits with no pattern to them, with some steps appearing normal. The consultant sits her on a chair, brings her right knee up, and notes that he can feel her left leg extend/exert force when he does this. What is the sign that the consultant has elucidated?

A.   Babinski's sign

B.   Hoover's sign

C.   Hoffman's sign

D.   Brudzinski's sign

E.   Lhermitte's sign

13.   A patient presents with an 8-month history of hearing loss. They have no other symptoms and no medical history. An audiogram shows globally reduced hearing in the left ear only, with an equal reduction in air and bone conduction. What is the best investigation to look for a possible cause?

A.   Repeat audiogram at 6 weeks

B.   CT head and neck scan

● C.   Pituitary MRI

D.   Cerebellopontine angle MRI

E.   Dix-Hallpike manoeuvre

14.   A 70-year-old female who is normally fit and well presents to the A&E complaining of sudden onset headache with blurred vision. It is the most painful headache she has ever had. She has hypertension and anxiety, and she is also on the neurosurgical waiting list for the removal of an acromegaly-causing pituitary adenoma. A CT scan shows an area of haemorrhage in the pituitary gland. What is the most likely diagnosis?

A.   Sheehan's syndrome

B.   Pituitary apoplexy

▲ C.   Subarachnoid haemorrhage

D.   Giant cell arteritis

E.   Empty sella syndrome

15.   A 43-year-old male is clerked into the A&E with suspected subarachnoid haemorrhage after suffering from a thunderclap headache whilst playing golf. An initial CT head scan was negative, so a lumbar puncture was arranged for 12 hours after symptom onset. What is most likely to be seen on the lumbar puncture if he does have a subarachnoid haemorrhage?

A.   Raised bilirubin levels

B.   Raised cerebrospinal fluid pressure

● C.   Raised lymphocyte count

D.   Raised neutrophil count

E.   Low cerebrospinal fluid glucose

16.   In the intensive care unit, you see a 32-year-old who was involved in a high-speed road traffic accident 3 days ago and has not been able to be weaned from ventilation. The critical care consultant explains to you that a provisional diagnosis of brainstem death is being considered. Which of the following tests can be used to indicate brainstem death?

A.   Presence of heart sounds

B.   Sluggish pupillary response

C.   Hypertension and bradycardia

D.   No response to pain stimuli

E.   Fixed and dilated pupils

17.   The clinical triad of pseudo-Argyll Robertson pupils, supranuclear gaze palsy, and convergence-retraction nystagmus best describes what?

A.   Tertiary syphilis

B.   Parinaud syndrome

C.   Holmes Adie pupil

D.   Marcus Gunn pupil

E.   Weber syndrome

18.   A 43-year-old lady presents with her extremely concerned husband. Over the last 2 months, she has experienced a steady decline in overall functioning. Previously a lawyer in a high stakes firm, she has been dismissed from her position due to her forgetting even the simplest of basic laws, and she can no longer attempt the crosswords that she used to be an expert in. Examination reveals myoclonus and severely impaired memory on the Montreal cognitive assessment test. What is the most likely diagnosis?

A.   Frontotemporal dementia

B.   Normal pressure hydrocephalus

C.   Creutzfeldt-Jakob Disease

D.   Encephalitis

E.   Depressive pseudodementia

19.   You are a medical student undertaking your fourth year GP placement when a patient presents with a headache. In her drug history, you note that she has been taking diazepam for anxiety for the last 20 years, and the GP is currently trying to slowly reduce her dose with the aim of eventually stopping it altogether. What is the action of this class of medication?

A.   Glutamate antagonist

B.   GABA antagonist

▲   C.   ACh receptor agonist

D.   GABA agonist

E.   Acetylcholinesterase inhibitor

20.   A patient presents to you with visual loss after a stroke. On examination, they have a right inferior quadrantanopia. What part of the brain is most likely affected to cause this visual loss?

A.   Left parietal lobe

B.   Left temporal lobe

▲   C.   Left optic nerve

D.   Right parietal lobe

E.   Right temporal lobe

21.   Whilst on a paediatrics rotation, you find a rather interesting case of a 9-year-old female who has presented with 3 distinct episodes of left arm weakness and slurred speech in the past year. An MRI scan reveals multiple areas of widespread infarcts across the brain. Apart from this, she is fit and well. She moved to the UK with her parents from Japan 5 years ago. What is the most likely diagnosis?

A.   CADASIL

B.   Muscular dystrophy

■   C.   Hurler syndrome

D.   Benign Rolandic epilepsy

E.   Moya Moya disease

22. A patient presents with a 6-week history of numbness and tingling in their feet. They have hypertension and a body mass index of 40. On examination, you note sensory loss in a stocking pattern on the feet, with several small ulcers present on the dorsum of the foot. The right foot also looks significantly deformed and concave in appearance. What is the most likely diagnosis?

    A. Subacute combined degeneration of the cord

    B. Syphilis

    C. Diabetic neuropathy

    D. Buerger's disease (Thromboangiitis obliterans)

    E. No pathological cause for their symptoms

23. A 14-year-old boy from a travelling family attends the GP with his parents. They describe him experiencing a gradual decline over the last 6 months, saying 'he has just not been himself'. He used to be at the top of his class, but now he has lost his ability to write and is displaying personality changes, becoming increasingly quiet and reserved when he used to be very bright and energetic. He has no allergies, was not vaccinated as a child, and his medical history is insignificant. His parents report that he suffered from a 'really bad bout' of measles when he was 2 years old. What is the most likely cause of his decline?

    A. Depression

    B. CNS lymphoma

    C. Creutzfeldt-Jakob disease

    D. Subacute Sclerosing panencephalitis

    E. Hypothyroidism

24. A patient presents with a 6-week history of double vision only when looking to the right, accompanied by progressive left-sided weakness. Where is the lesion?

    A. Cerebrum

    B. Midbrain

    C. Pons

    D. Medulla

    E. Spinal cord

25. A 29-year-old female presents to the A&E after a head injury following a road traffic accident. As an F1, you and the trauma team undertake an A-E assessment. You are asked by the consultant to assess her Glasgow Coma Scale (GCS). On examination, she opens her eyes to a painful stimulus, makes incomprehensible sounds, and localises to pain. What is the GCS you should tell the A&E consultant?

   A. 7
   B. 8
   ● C. 9
   D. 10
   E. 11

26. The parents of a 3-year-old boy bring him to see a local paediatric consultant. They are struggling with his intractable epilepsy, having tried 4 different anticonvulsant medications without success. He is also struggling in nursery, and the teacher has said that he is well behind his peers. On examination, it is clear that he has global developmental delay, and you notice a roughened patch of skin over the lumbar area of the back. What is the most likely diagnosis?

   A. Tuberous sclerosis
   B. West syndrome
   ■ C. Global developmental delay
   D. Rett syndrome
   E. Juvenile myoclonic epilepsy

27. A patient presents to the A&E with an acute episode of migraine. They are demanding treatment as they say the pain is unbearable. What is the best management plan?

   A. Topiramate
   B. Propranolol
   ● C. Sumatriptan
   D. Domperidone PO
   E. Simple analgesics

28.   James, a 44-year-old patient with known HIV and subsequent AIDS, presents
        with a 6-month history of general decline. He has developed progressive weakness
        affecting his left arm and leg, is very clumsy when he walks, and has double vision.
        His last CD4+ count done 2 weeks ago comes back as 30 cells/mm³. An MRI scan
        reveals bilateral white matter and thalamic lesions. What is the most likely
        diagnosis?

        A.   Primary CNS lymphoma

        B.   Progressive multifocal leukoencephalopathy

        C.   Creutzfeldt-Jakob disease

        D.   Subacute combined degeneration of the cord

        E.   Frontotemporal dementia

29.   Samira, a 31-year-old female, presents to her GP complaining of a lack of periods
        ever since the birth of her second child 8 months ago. Her first child was born
        without complications. In her notes, you find that she had suffered a significant
        post-partum haemorrhage after delivering her second child and required several
        blood transfusions. What is the most likely cause of her amenorrhoea?

        A.   Psychological amenorrhoea

        B.   Menopause

        C.   Infarction of the pituitary gland

        D.   Hypothalamic lesion

        E.   Meningioma

30.   In a patient with status epilepticus, what is the first line management?

        A.   Buccal midazolam 10 mg

        B.   Intravenous lorazepam 4 mg

        C.   Rectal diazepam 10 mg

        D.   Intramuscular glucagon 2 mg

        E.   Do nothing until directed by a senior

31.   Assuming no contraindications, what is the first line treatment (besides simple
        analgesics) for the prevention of migraine?

        A.   Topiramate

        B.   Verapamil

        C.   Diltiazem

        D.   Propranolol

        E.   Nimodipine

32.   A patient with a provisional diagnosis of Parkinson's also complains of frequent falls after rising from a sitting position, erectile dysfunction, and vomiting after food. What is the most likely cause?

A.   Multiple systems atrophy

B.   Corticobasal degeneration

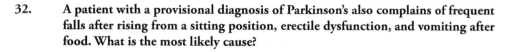

C.   Parkinson's and depression

D.   Parkinson's and dementia

E.   Progressive supranuclear palsy

33.   What MRC grade of power is assigned to a limb that has 'active movement against gravity' but not against resistance?

A.   1

B.   2

C.   3

D.   4

E.   5

34.   A 23-year-old female professional skateboarder is admitted to the A&E with a reduced consciousness level. She had a nasty crash two hours ago during a skateboarding event, where she reportedly lost consciousness for a few minutes but recovered and was able to continue the event. However, 2 hours later she deteriorated quickly. What is the most likely diagnosis?

A.   Skull fracture

B.   Hydrocephalus

C.   Acute subdural haematoma

D.   Acute extradural haematoma

E.   Scalp haematoma

35.   A 55-year-old female presents to her GP with a 6-week history of headache and worsening balance. She has a past medical history of depression and irritable bowel syndrome, and she underwent a mastectomy 2 years ago for breast cancer. She consumes 30 units of alcohol a week. What is the most likely diagnosis?

A.   Glioblastoma

B.   Medulloblastoma

C.   Multiple sclerosis

D.   Cerebral metastases

E.   Cerebellar degeneration due to alcohol abuse

36.   Which of the following is not a relative contraindication to a Lumbar puncture?

     A.   CT head scan shows a space-occupying lesion

     B.   Hypertension and bradycardia

     C.   Meningitis

     D.   Cardiovascular instability

     E.   Known coagulopathy

37.   A patient presents to the A&E with leg weakness that occurred suddenly without warning 4 hours ago, affecting both legs. She has also not been able to pass urine or feel the urge to urinate during this period. She has a history of stage 4 breast cancer. What is the best immediate management plan?

     A.   Lie upright, intravenous prednisolone

     B.   Lie flat, dexamethasone

     C.   Urgent oncology referral

     D.   Expectant management

     E.   Intravenous antibiotics

38.   What medication is used in subarachnoid haemorrhage to prevent the complication of cerebral vasospasm?

     A.   Verapamil

     B.   Lidocaine

     C.   Phenytoin

     D.   Nimodipine

     E.   Enalapril

39. A 73-year-old male attends the A&E department accompanied by his carer, who states that he has been more confused as of late and has been falling repeatedly. A CT head scan is shown below:

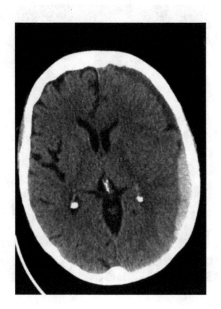

Based on the imaging, what is the most likely diagnosis?

A. Acute extradural haematoma

B. Basal skull fracture

C. Chronic subdural haematoma

D. Acute on chronic subdural haematoma

E. Acute subdural haematoma

40.   A patient attends their GP with a 4-week history of headache, which is progressively getting worse. An outpatient MRI head scan is shown below:

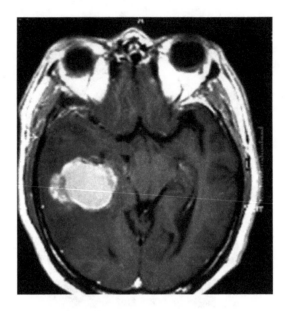

Based on the imaging, what is the most likely diagnosis?

A.   Foreign body

B.   Cerebral abscess

C.   Space-occupying lesion

D.   Acute ischaemia

E.   Hydrocephalus

ANSWERS

Practice Paper 1 — Answers

1) Correct answer: D

Pretty much a case of rote learning for this one — the classical triad of raised intracranial pressure is hypertension, bradycardia, and irregular respiration. The reasons behind this are complicated and not worth knowing. Ptosis, miosis, and facial anhidrosis are associated with Horner's syndrome, and supranuclear gaze palsy, pseudo Argyll Robertson pupils, and nystagmus are associated with Parinaud syndrome, which is due to a midbrain (brainstem) lesion such as a pineal gland tumour.

2) Correct answer: D

This would be correct as the diagnosis is a chronic subdural haematoma. This means that blood will not be acute, which would be in keeping with answer B, as the patient described in answer B fell 4 hours ago, representing an acute presentation. A refers to a classical acute extradural haematoma, while C is a subarachnoid haemorrhage which commonly occurs with exertion, neck stiffness from presence of blood in the cerebrospinal fluid, and subsequent meningeal irritation. Hence, D would be the answer as chronic subdural haematoma can classically present with intermittent confusion and should be considered in any elderly patient with a history of falls and/or who is on anticoagulation. E is describing an acute stroke.

3) Correct answer: E

CT scan head within 1 hour is the most appropriate initial management because the patient, although seemingly healthy, has features of a basal skull fracture, including bruising behind the mastoid process ('Battle's sign') and cerebrospinal fluid rhinorrhoea (clear nasal discharge). The other signs of a basal skull fracture are haemotympanum (blood in the ear) and panda/raccoon eyes (periorbital bruising). Patients with any of these signs after a head injury need to undergo a CT scan within 1 hour.

Indications to do a CT within 1 hour after a head injury are worth learning and they include:

GCS <13
GCS <15 2 hours after the injury
Signs of a basal skull fracture (as above)
Focal neurological deficit
Vomiting more than one time
Seizures after the head injury

Indications for CT head scan within 8 hours of injury include:
Anyone over the age of 65
People on anticoagulant or blood thinning medication such as warfarin
Dangerous mechanism of injury or fall from height
Source: NICE Head Injury Guidelines (2014).

4) Correct answer: C

This is a classical presentation of idiopathic intracranial hypertension (IIH) — signs of raised ICP but no lesion identified on the CT scan and visual acuity changes are also common in IIH for young obese females. The classic symptoms are headache, transient or persistent vision loss, pulsatile tinnitus (whooshing sound in the ears), and/or diplopia.

IIH can be diagnosed using a lumbar puncture, which may show raised cerebrospinal fluid pressure, or magnetic resonance venography to rule out other causes. The best treatment for IIH is simply weight loss, and a loss of 10–15% body weight has been shown to improve symptoms. Other options include acetazolamide, a carbonic anhydrase inhibitor that decreases cerebrospinal fluid production, and cerebrospinal fluid diversion via a ventriculoperitoneal shunt in refractory cases or if visual loss is a concern.

Glioblastoma would be visible on most CT head scans, is more common in older adults, and would most likely have neurological deficits, while cavernous sinus thrombosis would present with multiple cranial nerve defects (including III, IV, V1 and V2), and there is no head injury to suggest chronic subdural haematoma.

5) Correct answer: D

This lady has recently been given thrombolysis, with the biggest potential risk of doing so causing a bleed in the brain — also known as a haemorrhagic transformation. This is the most likely explanation as infarcted tissue is most likely to bleed, and any patient that displays an altered GCS or reduced consciousness level after thrombolysis requires an immediate CT head scan to rule out haemorrhagic transformation of the infarct. Malignant MCA syndrome would show a widespread infarct in the MCA territory during a CT scan (this patient's scan was normal), and subarachnoid haemorrhage, hypoglycaemia, and overuse of opiate medication would not be reasons for thrombolysis or the presentation.

6) Correct answer: D

The correct answer here is a cerebral (brain) abscess, because the patient has presented with fever, raised intracranial pressure, focal neurological deficits and confusion. The patient also has had a recent episode of sinusitis, which if bacterial, can rarely spread to the CNS causing a cerebral abscess. Other risk factors include recent neurosurgical intervention such as surgeries that can introduce infection, ENT infections (such as sinusitis, mastoiditis, or otitis media), endocarditis (from fragments or vegetations embolising to the brain), intravenous drug use, or being immunocompromised. Imaging such as CT or MRI scans (MRI is preferred for making the diagnosis) can outline ring-enhancing lesions that are often well circumscribed. The ring-enhancing nature often discriminates this from tumours, which may be less well formed.

Management involves urgent referral to a neurosurgery unit for advice and guidance, with usual treatment being a prolonged course of broad spectrum intravenous antibiotics. The triad of fever, headache, and focal neurological signs should make you think of a possible cerebral abscess in an exam question.

Source: Eureka! Neurology and Neurosurgery (2016)

7) Correct answer: C

This gentleman has the classical features of neuropathic pain, most likely due to his poorly controlled diabetes. Amitriptyline is frequently utilised as a first line agent for neuropathic pain. However, he also has BPH, and giving amitriptyline in this scenario could precipitate urinary retention due to its antimuscarinic effects and should be avoided here. Pregabalin and gabapentin are similar agents to the GABA inhibitory receptor and are commonly used for neuropathic pain and anxiety. Duloxetine is a serotonin and noradrenaline reuptake inhibitor and is used as an antidepressant and for neuropathic pain (DUALoxetine: blocks two transmitters, used for 2 conditions). Paracetamol is not commonly used for neuropathic pain specifically.

A stepwise approach to neuropathic pain (NICE guidelines) are outlined below:

1. Amitriptyline, duloxetine, gabapentin, or pregabalin as initial treatment
2. If initial treatment not effective, switch to a different drug
3. Consider capsaicin cream for people with localised neuropathic pain who wish to avoid, or who cannot tolerate, oral treatments.

8) Correct answer: C

The Glasgow Coma Scale (GCS) is a quick and frequently utilised assessment of consciousness level, is very examinable, and should be learned by heart. It is categorised into eye (E), verbal (V), and motor (M) responses, with all three combined to make a total score out of 15. Eye responses have a maximum score of 4, verbal a maximum score of 5, and motor a maximum score of 6 (EVM-456). A key point of the GCS is that you should score the patient's BEST response (i.e., if they score higher on one arm compared to the other, the higher score should be used). The GCS is outlined in the table below. A tricky one to remember is that withdrawal from the pain stimulus scores 4 points, and groaning (or incomprehensible sounds) scores 2 points.

Glasgow Coma Scale		
Feature	**Response**	**Score**
Eye	Open spontaneously	4
	Open to voice	3
	Open to pain	2
	No eye opening	1
Verbal	Orientated	5
	Confused	4
	Inappropriate words	3
	Incomprehensible sounds	2
	No verbal response	1
Motor	Obeys commands	6
	Localising pain	5
	Withdrawal from pain	4
	Flexion to pain	3
	Extension to pain	2
	No motor response	1

9) Answer: B

The correct answer is B. Horner's syndrome is caused by damage to the sympathetic innervation of the eye (which can happen at 3 levels) and classically gives a triad of ptosis (drooping or falling of the upper eyelid), miosis (small or constricted pupil), and ipsilateral facial anhidrosis (lack of sweating on the same side of the face as the lesion). There may also be enophthalmos (posterior displacement of the eyeball). First-order neurons in the pathway come from the hypothalamus and brainstem, second-order neurons enter the cervical sympathetic nervous system chain, and third-order neurons return up the neck to innervate the eye. Causes of Horner's syndrome are remembered at the level of the dysfunction where they occur and are outlined in the table below (with Pancoast tumours [apical lung tumours] being the most commonly asked about in exams!):

Location	Causes
Brain and brainstem	Massive cerebral infarction Lateral medullary syndrome
T1 root	Apical lung tumour (Pancoast tumour) Cervical rib
Sympathetic chain/carotid artery	Carotid artery dissection After thyroid/carotid/laryngeal surgery
Miscellaneous	Cluster headache (usually temporary)

Diagnosis is based on clinical signs and treatment is usually related to identifying the cause, such as treating lung cancer if a Pancoast tumour is the cause.

Ataxia, ophthalmoplegia, and confusion describe the triad for Wernicke's encephalopathy, which is caused by acute thiamine (vitamin B1) deficiency, while headache, fever, and altered consciousness level describe encephalitis.

10) Correct Answer: E

This lady is presenting with classical symptoms of a subarachnoid haemorrhage, and this should be urgently ruled out. The most appropriate initial investigation is a non-contrast CT head scan, which can detect 95% of subarachnoid haemorrhages within 6 hours of symptom onset. If this is normal, a lumbar puncture should be requested at 12 hours after the headache onset. The classic sign on lumbar puncture of a subarachnoid haemorrhage is xanthochromia, a yellow appearance of cerebrospinal fluid due to the presence of bilirubin, a breakdown product of red blood cells that have got into cerebrospinal fluid due to the bleed. Another (more subtle) sign of subarachnoid haemorrhage is raised cerebrospinal fluid pressure (see the cerebrospinal fluid interpretation table on Page 153).

If the cause of a subarachnoid haemorrhage is suspected to be from rupture of an aneurysm, a CT angiography is often requested to test for this once the patient is stable, which can help delineate to the blood vessels involved in a possible aneurysm.

11) Correct answer: A

This is a classical diagnosis of motor neurone disease, the most common of which is called amyotrophic lateral sclerosis. This typically presents as an elderly male patient (it is more common in males) with progressive weakness, swallowing difficulties, and general decline. On examination, you will typically find a combination of upper and lower motor neuron signs, such as wasting, fasciculation coupled with brisk reflexes, and clonus (for more upper and motor neuron signs, see Paper 1, Question 28, Page 10). To diagnose, the patient needs clinical, electrophysical, or neuropathologic evidence of both left and upper motor neuron degeneration, as well as evidence of progressive spread within a region or to other body regions. The condition presents insidiously and is incurable. Riluzole, a drug designed to block glutamatergic transmission (thought to be involved in the disease process leading to damage of neurones), only improves survival by a few months and most patients unfortunately die within 3–5 years, mostly due to complications around ventilation (e.g., respiratory failure) or dysphagia and subsequent malnutrition/aspiration.

12) Correct answer: D

The triad for normal pressure hydrocephalus (NPH) can be remembered as **w**et, **w**acky, and **w**obbly, or urinary incontinence, dementia/memory impairment, and gait ataxia/falls. This is an important cause of potentially reversible dementia and needs to be identified quickly. See Paper 3, Question 28, Page 41 for a description of NPH and its management.

13) Correct answer: D

The most common primary cause of brain metastases is bronchial (lung) carcinoma, which accounts for almost 50% of all brain metastases, followed by breast cancer (15%), melanoma (10%), and colon cancer (5%). The most common causes of brain metastases are shown below:

Primary site	%
Lung	50
Breast	15
Melanoma	10
Colon	5
Other	20

Any patient with a known malignancy and new onset headache or progressive neurological symptoms or decline needs an urgent CT or MRI head scan to rule out metastasis. Treatment is with dexamethasone to acutely reduce cerebral oedema (swelling around the tumour) and referral to neurosurgery services to consider surgical removal if appropriate. If surgery is not appropriate due to comorbidities or patient choice, radiotherapy or stereotactic radiosurgery — a more targeted type of radiotherapy — can be considered.

Source: Davidson's Principles and Practice of Medicine, 24th Edition (2018)

14) Correct answer: E

A lumbar puncture is a useful way to test for multiple conditions such as meningitis, intracranial hypertension, and subarachnoid haemorrhage. A needle is inserted into the subarachnoid space with the patient in the left lateral decubitus position (lying down on the left-hand side) and cerebrospinal fluid is withdrawn and sampled. The most severe (although rare) risk of doing a lumbar puncture is the risk of coning, where pressure changes during needle insertion cause parts of the brain to 'herniate' down towards the medulla, putting pressure on the brain's respiratory centres and causing respiratory arrest. This is life-threatening and should be avoided. The most common reasons for coning include raised intracranial pressure from mass lesions such as tumours and other space-occupying lesions, and thus it is important to rule these out before proceeding.

If in doubt, request a CT head scan BEFORE doing a lumbar puncture to rule out raised intracranial pressure. The following are absolute contraindications to performing a lumbar puncture, and for finals you should know at least 2 of them:

> - Bradycardia and hypertension, papilloedema, unequal or dilated pupils
> - Reduced level of consciousness (GCS <9)
> - Shock
> - Coagulation abnormalities
> - Cardiovascular or respiratory compromise/insufficiency
> - Focal neurological signs (e.g., weakness)
> - Local infection at the lumbar puncture site

Source: NICE Meningitis (Bacterial) and Meningococcal Septicaemia in Under 16s: Recognition, Diagnosis and Management (2015)

15) Correct answer: A

The correct answer is sodium valproate, which is associated with weight gain and hair loss (which then grows back curlier!) and is highly teratogenic — it is associated with neural tube defects, so this medication should be <u>avoided</u> in women of childbearing age. The side effects of commonly used anticonvulsant medications are outlined below:

Medication	Indications	Side effects
Sodium valproate	Generalised seizures Partial seizures	Weight gain Reversible hair loss Teratogenic
Carbamazepine	Focal seizures Generalised tonic-clonic seizures	CYP450 Inducer (can reduce efficacy of combined oral contraceptive pills) Hyponatraemia
Phenytoin	Not used much anymore — can be used for focal/tonic-clonic second line treatment for status epilepticus (after lorazepam) Prevention and treatment of seizures during or following neurosurgery or head injury	Gingival (gum) hypertrophy, acne, and hirsutism with long term use
Lamotrigine	Focal seizures (first line monotherapy)	Headache, drowsiness, **skin rash** (needs urgent review)
Levetiracetam (Keppra®)	Focal seizures (first line monotherapy if carbamazepine or lamotrigine not tolerated) Add on therapy for myoclonic or generalised tonic-clonic seizures	Minimal drug interactions (compared to other antiepileptic drugs), NOT teratogenic Confusion, sedation, behavioural change in children Mood disturbance and psychiatric effects uncommon

Source: The Top 100 Drugs: Clinical Pharmacology and Practical Prescribing (2018)

16) Correct answer: C

Cluster headache is the correct diagnosis, because cluster headache is more common in males (6:1 male-female ratio), the headache lasts 2 hours (cluster headaches typically last between 15 minutes and 3 hours) whereas migraines typically last for 4–72 hours, and the patient has restlessness during the episodes given that he cannot stay still and walks around — a migraine patient will want to stay still and may have photophobia (lights appearing very bright causing disturbance) and excessive tearing (autonomic symptoms are common with cluster headache). Examination and ophthalmoscopy are normal, which rules out a space-occupying lesion, and there is no medication history, so it is unlikely that he has medication overuse headache. The key differences you need to know between headache types for exams is outlined below:

Type	Duration	Triggers	Clinical features	Treatment (acute)	Treatment (chronic)
Migraine	4–72 hours	Foods (e.g., chocolate, cheese, wine)	Female Photophobia Visual disturbance (scotoma and fortification spectre) Phonophobia (fear of sounds/noises)	Any of: Paracetamol Aspirin Metoclopramide/ Domperidone (if nausea present) Triptans	First line: Propranolol or topiramate Second line: Antidepressants (amitriptyline) Third line/ resistant: Greater occipital nerve block Botulinum toxin type A
Cluster headache	15 minutes– 3 hours	Alcohol	Male (3:1) Restlessness Autonomic symptoms (e.g., red eye, lacrimation) 'Alarm clock' headache — wakes patient up and occurs at the same time each day	First line: High flow O$_2$ + Subcutaneous triptans (5HT agonists, e.g., sumatriptan)	Verapamil Lithium
Tension headache	30 minutes– 1 week	Dehydration Stress Inappropriate prescription lenses	Bilateral 'band-like' pain around the head Mild to moderate Non-pulsatile No nausea and vomiting	Not usually required	Simple analgesia (e.g., paracetamol) Avoid opioids and frequent drugs due to medication overuse headaches

(*Continued*)

Type	Duration	Triggers	Clinical features	Treatment (acute)	Treatment (chronic)
Medication overuse headache	Variable	Withdrawal from medications	Headache worse despite medications More medication increases do not resolve the headache Long history of taking medications	Not treated acutely	Gradually withdraw pain medications
Raised intracranial pressure headache	Subacute (weeks to months)	Coughing, sneezing, bending down	Worse in mornings Blurred/double vision, may have weakness	Dexamethasone to reduce cerebral oedema and intracranial pressure	Urgent 2-week referral if malignancy/space-occupying lesion suspected

Source: Eureka! Neurology and Neurosurgery (2016)

17) Correct answer: E

This patient has a classic case of trigeminal neuralgia, thought to be caused by compression of the trigeminal nerve by a branch of the superior cerebellar artery. Patients present just like this one — with excruciating facial pain (they may describe this as the worst pain they have ever had) and extreme sensitivity (the featured exam buzzword is that shaving, brushing teeth, and even the wind can trigger pain). The pain is sharp, stabbing, and electric shock-like in nature. It was historically known as 'suicide disease' because the severity of pain often drove those afflicted to end their own life.

The first line treatment for trigeminal neuralgia is carbamazepine, which reduces the firing of nerve impulses that generates the pain. If carbamazepine is contraindicated or not effective, a specialist neurology referral is required. Other approaches include using other drugs such as Gabapentin and Lamotrigine, and refractory cases can be managed with surgical decompression or balloon compression.

18) Correct answer: D

As explained above, the first line treatment for trigeminal neuralgia is carbamazepine. Propranolol is used for the prevention of migraine, primidone is used as a treatment for benign essential tremor, sodium valproate is used for generalised seizures, and lithium is used occasionally as a second line treatment (after verapamil) for cluster headache.

19) Correct answer: E

This patient has a suspected acute onset stroke, so an immediate non-contrast CT head scan should be arranged. This is to rule out a brain bleed or any other contraindications, as the patient may be eligible for thrombolysis, a clot-busting intravenous treatment that can improve prognosis if given quickly enough (for thrombolysis criteria see Paper 2, Question 10, Page 20). However, it is important to first rule out hypoglycaemia as this can potentially cause symptoms that mimic a stroke. This is especially important in this case as he is currently taking gliclazide, an oral hypoglycaemic agent, for his diabetes. A capillary blood glucose performed within seconds can quickly rule this out and therefore would be the first investigation to carry out in the A&E department as part of an A–E assessment. Other important stroke mimics can be remembered by the **4 S's**: **s**eizures, **s**epsis, **s**yncope, and **s**ugar (hypoglycaemia).

20) Correct answer: A

This child has Infantile spasms (also known as West syndrome), a childhood epilepsy syndrome. Infantile spasms are most common among children aged 3–12 months and involve 'salaam' attacks — violent flexor spasms of the head, neck, and arms followed by hyperextension and drawing up of the knees to the chest (this sometimes resemble colic). An electroencephalogram may reveal the classic exam buzzword of 'hypsarrhythmia' — chaotic and irregular high amplitude waves. It is associated with tuberous sclerosis. Treatment is with vigabatrin or steroids, and prognosis is poor. The childhood epilepsy syndromes are summarised in the table below:

Diagnosis	Key features	EEG findings	Treatments
Infantile spasms (West syndrome)	'Salaam' attacks (flexion of limbs followed by hyperextension) 3–12 months old Resembles colic	Hypsarrhythmia	Vigabatrin, steroids
Benign Rolandic epilepsy (epilepsy with centrotemporal spikes)	4–10 years old Tonic-clonic seizures in sleep OR Simple focal- abnormal feelings in the tongue and face	Centrotemporal spikes (in Rolandic area)	Remits in adolescence, no treatment required
Panayiotopoulos syndrome (early onset benign occipital epilepsy)	1–5 years old Autonomic seizures: vomiting, unresponsive staring in sleep Head and eye deviation	Posterior sharp waves, occipital discharges	Remits in childhood
Juvenile myoclonic epilepsy	10–20 years old Triad of seizure types: Myoclonic, generalised tonic-clonic and absence Worse after wakening 'knocking drinks/cereal' — classic feature Worse after alcohol or sleep deprivation	3–6 Hz generalised 'spike and wave' discharge	Needs indefinite antiepileptic medication (sodium valproate or lamotrigine)

(Continued)

Diagnosis	Key features	EEG findings	Treatments
Blue breath holding spells	Under 3 years old Hold breath when upset or angry = go blue and lose consciousness	n/a	Conservative
Reflex asystolic syncope (reflex anoxic seizure)	6 months–2 years Triggered by head trauma, pain/cold Vagal-induced cardiac asystole = syncope +/– jerks	n/a	Conservative
Febrile convulsions	Fever + seizures in any child 6 months–5 years old	n/a	Antipyretics (but does not reduce seizure risk) — many recur Reassurance

21) Correct answer: B

This patient has Wernicke's aphasia, also known as receptive dysphasia. Both aphasia and dysphasia refer to problems with speaking and are often used interchangeably. The Wernicke's area is located in the left temporal lobe and is responsible for understanding and processing what other people say to us, whilst the Broca's area is located in the left frontal lobe and is situated on the left-hand side for about 90% of right-handed people and 70% of left-handed people. Broca's is responsible for controlling the muscles of speech that enable us to talk. Therefore, if Wernicke's is damaged but the Broca's area is intact, a patient will be able to talk fluently but have impaired comprehension. That is, they will not be able to understand dialogue or questions asked, so speech will be jumbled and not make sense. For Broca's, patients are able to understand what they are being asked but cannot articulate themselves, so they are often frustrated at their inability to do so. The most common cause of both Broca's and Wernicke's dysphasia is stroke. Conduction aphasia refers to damage to the articulate fasciculus, which connects the two areas together. Damage to this area causes impaired repetition (for some reason!), so a patient with preserved Broca's and Wernicke's areas would not be able to repeat words that are asked of them. Dysarthria is damage to the muscles involved in articulating speech without higher involvement (e.g., tongue muscles), and dysphagia is difficulty with swallowing.

∗Source: *StatPearls: Conduction Aphasia (2020)*

22) Correct answer: C

Carpal tunnel syndrome is caused by compression of the median nerve, often by the flexor retinaculum (a band above the carpal tunnel). It is more common in females and patients with hypothyroidism, rheumatoid arthritis, pregnancy, and acromegaly. There is no known association with multiple sclerosis. The patient classically presents with wrist pain that is worse at night, described as a shooting pain and/or numbness, tingling, or a 'funny feeling', and is often relieved by shaking the arm over the bed ('wake and shake'). Examination may reveal wasting of the thenar eminence (muscles over the thumb supplied by the median nerve) and a positive Tinel's (**T**inel's = **T**ap-tapping over the wrist causes numbness/paraesthesia in the thenar eminence and lateral side of the hand) and Phalen's test (flexing the wrist for 30 seconds recreates symptoms). Management strategies include conservative with pain relief, wrist splinting at night, steroid injections, and then surgical decompression if refractory to these treatments. Wasting of the thenar eminence is also an indication for surgical decompression (see Paper 4, Question 23, Page 149 for a table comparing the common nerve compressions).

23) Correct answer: B

Wernicke's encephalopathy is caused by acute deficiency of the vitamin thiamine (vitamin B1). Patients at risk are most notably those with alcohol misuse, malnutrition, and excessive vomiting (it can rarely occur in hyperemesis gravidarum during pregnancy). It presents with the classic clinical triad of confusion, ataxia, and ophthalmoplegia (limited eye movements or difficulty initiating eye movements). The acute treatment is with Pabrinex®, consisting of vitamin B replacement (most importantly vitamin B1) and a long-acting benzodiazepine such as chlordiazepoxide to control agitation, and often co-existing with alcohol withdrawal. Wernicke's encephalopathy is reversible and the main aim of treatment is to prevent the irreversible complication of Korsakoff's psychosis — irreversible anterograde amnesia with confabulation (falsification of events because the patient cannot remember them due to the degeneration of mamillary bodies involved in the memory circuits of the brain).

Of note, the triad of diarrhoea, dementia, and dermatitis (also known as Casal's necklace) is characteristic of niacin (vitamin B3) deficiency.

24) Correct answer: A

This patient has Charcot-Marie-Tooth disease, also known as hereditary motor and sensory neuropathy, which is a group of autosomal dominant inherited peripheral neuropathies that causes demyelination or axon loss, followed by 'onion skin' regeneration of nerves. This leads to the classical syndrome of distal muscle weakness (most usually in the lower limbs like the foot, tibia, and peroneal groups), leading to an 'inverted champagne bottle' appearance, variable loss of sensation and reflexes, and pes cavus (a deformed, concave-shaped foot) or hammer toes. It often presents in children or in early adulthood. Diagnosis can be confirmed by family history and neurophysiology studies showing reduced motor conduction velocity in affected areas. There are two types of Charcot-Marie-Tooth disease, but it is very unlikely that you will need to know their differences for medical finals.

Other causes of peripheral neuropathies include diabetic neuropathy, chronic alcoholism, nutritional deficiencies such as vitamin B12 deficiency, Guillain-Barré syndrome, trauma/ injury, and peripheral neuropathy is secondary to drugs such as chemotherapy.

Source: Kumar and Clark's Clinical Medicine, 10th Edition (2020)

25) Correct answer: C

Dermatomes are easily examinable (even for medical finals) and easy to forget, so It's important to stay on top of them as a clinical medical student. The little finger is supplied by Dermatome C8. C6 supplies the thumb and the first 1.5 fingers, and the middle finger is supplied by C7. The key dermatomes for the upper limb are shown in the table below:

Body part	Dermatome
Back of head	C2
Clavicles	C4
Regimental badge area	C5
Thumb	C6
Tip of index finger	C7
Tip of little finger	C8
Anterior/medial elbow	T1
Underneath armpit	T2
Nipple line	T4

26) Correct answer: C

The sign being elicited is called Hoffman's sign and it is exactly as described in this question: you hold the patient's hand and flick the nail of the middle finger, and if it is positive, the thumb and index finger will spontaneously contract. A positive Hoffman's sign is an indication of an upper motor neuron or corticospinal cause of pathology, such as cervical cord compression secondary to degenerative cervical myelopathy (see Paper 2, Question 23, Page 24). Babinski's sign is indicated by curling of the big toe upward and not downward when an object is rolled up the sole of the foot, which is indicative of an upper motor neuron lesion. Hoover's sign is when flexing one knee from a flexed position causes the contralateral knee to extend — this is often used to diagnose functional neurological disorders. Brudzinski's sign is when you flex the neck, which causes automatic flexion of the hips and knees and is indicative of meningitis, and Lhermitte's sign is pain and paraesthesia — similar to electric shocks moving down the arms and legs after neck flexion, and is positive in multiple sclerosis. These signs are summarised in the table below:

Sign name	How do you test it?	What does it indicate?
Babinski's sign	Roll a non-sharp object from bottom to the top of the sole of the foot Positive if the big toe extends (should normally flex)	Upper motor neuron pathology (e.g., Stroke, tumour, multiple sclerosis)
Hoover's sign	Have a patient lying down and flex the non-affected (weak) leg Normally the non-affected leg should extend; if absent, the sign is positive	Functional neurological disorders (e.g., conversion disorders)
Hoffman's sign	Hold patient's arm, flick the middle finger Positive if there is spontaneous contraction of the thumb and index finger	Upper motor neuron lesion at cervical spine level (e.g., degenerative cervical myelopathy)
Brudzinski's sign	Neck flexion causes involuntary flexion of hips and knees	Meningitis
Kernig's sign	Flex hip at knee and knee at hip, then straighten leg Positive if neck stiffness occurs	Meningeal irritation (mostly meningitis), subarachnoid haemorrhage
Lhermitte's sign	Neck flexion causes 'electric shocks' down the trunk and limbs	Multiple sclerosis, degenerative cervical myelopathy

27) Correct answer: C

This is a classic diagnosis of idiopathic Parkinson's disease. The patient has almost all of the hallmark features, the core of which can be remembered using the mnemonic 'TRAP': **T**remor, **R**igidity (like a lead pipe), **A**kinesia (or bradykinesia — slowness of movements), and **P**ostural instability. The tremor appears at rest, is better with movement (in contrast to a benign essential tremor where the tremor appears or is made worse on movement), and is usually 3–7 Hz (3–7 shakes per second). Other features include loss of smell (anosmia — very commonly reported as the first symptom!), micrographia (small, illegible handwriting), and reduced facial expression (described as mask-like facies or, more correctly, hypomimia). Depression, urinary problems, and dementia are also common in the condition. All suspected cases of Parkinson's disease should be referred urgently to a neurologist specialising in movement disorders BEFORE commencing treatment — this is to allow confirmation of diagnosis and initiation of specialist treatments (discussed later in the book). There are no features in this case to indicate Parkinson's plus syndrome (Paper 2, Question 1, Page 17).

28) Correct answer: D

A positive Babinski's sign (movement of the big toe upwards when dragging an object from the heel towards the top of the big toe) is suggestive of an upper motor neuron lesion, which indicates damage to the brain, higher centres, or central spinal cord, whereas a lower motor neuron lesion indicates damage to the distal nerves that directly connect to muscles. A summary of the two signs is shown below — seeing both upper and lower motor neuron signs on examination almost always indicates motor neurone disease.

Upper motor neuron sign	Lower motor neuron sign
Weakness	Weakness
No muscle wasting	Muscle wasting
Clonus (rhythmic contractions evoked by a sudden stretch of muscle and tendon) — most tested on the ankle	Fasciculations
Hypertonia	Hypotonia
Brisk/normal reflexes	Diminished/absent reflexes
Spasticity: 'Spastic catch' or 'clasp-knife' phenomenon*	

Spastic catch: limb 'catches' with spasticity suddenly on movement, leading to abrupt stop.

Clasp knife: rapid, sudden decrease in resistance when trying to flex a joint.

*Source: Macleod's Clinical Examination, 14th Edition (2018)

29) Correct answer: B

The sudden nature of the presentation after a fall suggests an acute pathology. The diagnosis is an acute subdural haematoma. This is caused by the rupture of bridging veins in the subdural space in response to trauma. The two main risk factors are increased age and alcohol abuse (both of which this patient has), leading to brain atrophy, stretching of the cerebral veins, and hence increased chances of rupture. It is important to know how this will look on a CT scan (as well as for descriptive purposes in an OSCE scenario): subdural haematomas are crescent, concave, or banana-shaped and cross suture lines. In contrast, an acute extradural haematoma will be convex or lens-shaped, will most likely not cross suture lines, and may often be associated with a parietal or temporal skull fracture. Identifying this difference is crucial and it is a very frequently asked question in exams.

An acute extradural haematoma is seen often in young patients after head trauma, such as a cricket ball hitting the side of the head. The patient may briefly lose consciousness before recovering completely — this is referred to as the 'lucid interval' — and then may quickly deteriorate due to swelling and raised intracranial pressure from the bleed occurring outside the dural space. The haematoma appears as a convex or lens-shaped hyperdensity (i.e., brighter or more white than the surrounding brain tissue).

A chronic subdural haematoma tends to present with intermittent confusion, often following a seemingly trivial head trauma, and the patient may have residual weakness on the opposite side of the head injury as well. Pneumocephalus simply refers to the presence of air inside the brain tissue, and more details are not likely required for medical students. It is most commonly encountered following trauma or surgery.

Basal skull fracture has been described in Paper 1, Question 3, Page 1.

Source: *Radiopaedia.org*

30) Correct answer: D

A rapidly enlarging head circumference over the 95th percentile in any infant requires at least an urgent (if not emergency) referral to a paediatrician or paediatric neurosurgical team. This is because the cause may be from hydrocephalus (enlarged ventricles in the brain), which can be due to serious causes such as brain tumours, brain bleeding (intraventricular haemorrhage is most common in neonates), and infections like meningitis. This patient has likely developed hydrocephalus secondary to intraventricular haemorrhage, the risk of which is increased in premature babies and should be considered the most likely diagnosis until indicated otherwise. Hydrocephalus leads to increased intracranial pressure, which can manifest with the following signs in infants specifically: bulging anterior fontanelle (as this has not yet closed in infants), enlarged head circumference or macrocephaly (microcephaly is a small head circumference and therefore is not a cause), dilated scalp veins, and 'sun-setting', whereby the infant continually looks down and cannot bring their eyes or eyebrows up. Diagnosis can be confirmed by cranial ultrasound if the fontanelle is open — this can help with identification of the enlarged ventricles. Treatment usually involves inserting a ventriculoperitoneal shunt — a device that drains excess accumulated cerebrospinal fluid from the ventricles into the abdomen — reducing ventricle size and intracranial pressure as a result.

31) Correct answer: A

This patient has somatisation disorder. Ectopic beats are generally a normal finding in the ECGs of healthy people, so there is no arrythmia. The patient is not seeking out a specific diagnosis such as cancer, which rules out hypochondrial disorder (hypochondriac = Cancer), and the patient does not appear to be inventing symptoms for the psychological gain of the sick role, ruling out Munchausen's.

Somatisation disorder involves a patient complaining of multiple symptoms affecting different body systems (this patient has cardiac, dermatological, genitourinary, and gastro symptoms), often over many years. The key to diagnosis is that the investigation results are NORMAL. Treatment is with reassurance, although this is often difficult to communicate to the patient.

Hypochondrial disorder is a fear of having a medical disorder (most commonly cancer) despite evidence to the contrary. The patient may refuse to accept medical assurance or normal investigations and demand more extensive tests. The fixation on a single condition or system is key here. The difference between hypochondrial and somatisation disorder can be remembered as **S**omatisation = **S**ymptoms, hypochondriac = **C**ancer.

Munchausen's syndrome is a factitious disorder where patients feign physical or psychological symptoms in order to receive medical attention and benefit from appearing sick.

Source: Psychiatry PRN: Principles, Reality, Next Steps (2020)

32) Correct answer: D

This patient has malignant spinal cord compression, most likely secondary to his advanced prostate cancer. Malignant spinal cord compression occurs in 3–5% of patients with cancer, with the most common cancer causes being multiple myeloma, followed by prostate, breast, and lastly lung cancer. 70% occur in the thoracic vertebrae (because there are more of them), with 20% in the lumbosacral region and 10% being cervical. It is a neurological emergency due to the potentially reversible risk of severe disability (quadriplegia/paraplegia) and loss of bowel or bladder function. It has a poor prognosis, with 30% survival at one year.

The typical symptoms are back pain 'like a band', particularly around the thoracic region, and symptoms of cauda equina syndrome (weakness, urinary/bowel incontinence, sexual dysfunction etc). Immediate management is crucial, and the following steps should be undertaken: the patient should be placed FLAT (not upright) and given a high-dose dexamethasone (16mg) to reduce swelling from the compression. Next, the patient should, depending on their previous functional status and comorbidities, be referred to neurosurgery for consideration of emergency surgical decompression, but in most cases calling the oncology team for urgent advice would be the best management after dexamethasone.

*Source: Oxford Handbook of Palliative Care, 3rd Edition (2019).

33) Correct answer: E

Oh Brown-Sequard syndrome — another 'you're never going to see it but it's a med school favourite' question. Caused by a spinal cord hemi-section, it can be remembered by the memory aid 'One leg weak and one leg numb' — On the Ipsilateral (same) side of the lesion/injury, you get impaired sensory transmission of the dorsal columns which supply proprioception and vibration, and you also get impaired motor transmission of the corticospinal tract, which causes weakness. On the side opposite the lesion (contralateral), you get impaired sensory transmission of the spinothalamic tract, which supplies pain and temperature. So putting this altogether, a lesion on the right hand side would cause:

Weakness on the right-hand side, with impaired proprioception and vibration and:

Loss of pain and temperature on the left-hand side.

The most common cause of Brown-Sequard syndrome Is trauma (typically from a stabbing/gunshot wound).

That's probably all you need to know.

Source: Crash Course Neurology, 2019

34) Correct answer: B

This patient has a right third cranial nerve palsy and has all the characteristic features: The eye is deviated in a 'down and out' fashion due to weakness of muscles that bring the eye up and centrally, the pupil is fixed, dilated, and unreactive to light because the parasympathetic part of the oculomotor nerve is responsible for pupil constriction in response to light, and there is a droopy eyelid because the oculomotor nerve supplies the levator palpebrae superioris muscle that elevates the eyelid.

The causes of third cranial nerve palsies are raised intracranial pressure from a space-occupying lesion such as a tumour, a posterior communicating aneurysm (which would classically cause a <u>painful</u> third cranial nerve palsy), and diabetes (results in only a partial third cranial nerve palsy as the pupil response is spared due to the diabetic microangiopathy not affecting the parasympathetic fibres affecting the pupil).

A fourth cranial nerve palsy often presents with double vision that is classically vertical (so two images are seen, one on top of the other), and when asked to look down and laterally, the eye would not be able to do so (in a third cranial nerve palsy, the eye goes down and out because the trochlear nerve muscles are free to act on their own). The most common cause is trauma.

An abducens nerve palsy presents with double vision, often occurring side by side, and when asked to move the eye laterally (looking to the side), the patient will be unable to do so as this is the function of the abducens nerve. It is commonly affected in raised intracranial pressure caused by anything, which is often referred to as a 'false localising sign' because although the sixth cranial nerve is affected, the cause of the problem could be anywhere in the brain and cause raised intracranial pressure.

The trigeminal nerve does not supply eye movement.

35) Correct answer: C

This young boy has Wilson's disease, an autosomal recessive disorder caused by deficiency of caeruloplasmin, which binds to copper. This leads to excess intracellular copper in the body, which most severely affects the liver, brain, and basal ganglia. The classical examination finding is the presence of a golden-brown ring (Keyser-Fleischer ring) during eye examination, which is pathognomonic. Patients can also present with signs of liver disease and liver failure if untreated.

Wilson's disease commonly presents with psychiatric complications in children, such as behavioural disturbance, memory problems, and even dementia. This patient displays all of these symptoms. Diagnosis is supported by a low caeruloplasmin level, elevated unbound serum copper, and high urinary copper excretion, while treatment is with copper-binding agents that facilitate its excretion (e.g., penicillamine) and is reversible in most cases.

There is no family history or chorea to suggest Huntington's disease (see Paper 2, Question 4, Page 18), the patient does not have a previous history of syphilis, and there is no mention of a previous measles infection or antivaccination history to suggest SSPE (Paper 5, Question 23, Page 70 — a rare but fatal long-term complication of measles infection).

36) Correct answer: B

This patient has acromegaly, which is caused by excess growth hormone secretion. Growth hormones make every tissue in the body grow, and you characteristically get a patient whose appearance has slowly changed over time, with increases in shoe and finger size being the classic changes. The patient may also have hypertension due to excess growth hormones and carpal tunnel syndrome from excessive tissue growth in the compartment. Patients can also get sleep apnoea from an enlarged tongue and tissues, which reduce the flow through the airway. Examination may reveal an enlarged tongue (macroglossia) and prognathism (protrusion of the lower jaw outwards). The most common cause of acromegaly is pituitary adenoma, which can grow enough to compress the optic chiasm and result in bitemporal hemianopia (tunnel vision — the outer visual fields are affected). Most students know this part, but it can also only cause the superior visual field to be affected. A cause of inferior bitemporal hemianopia is a craniopharyngioma (brain tumour derived from pituitary gland embryonic tissue), which would present in someone much younger (usually a child) and with growth disturbance.

The causes of different visual field losses that you need to know for exams are summarised in this table:

Visual loss	Location	Causes	Diagram of eyes (with loss)
Unilateral blindness	Optic nerve	Brain tumours	
Bitemporal hemianopia	Optic chiasm	Superior: pituitary adenoma Inferior: craniopharyngioma	
Homonymous hemianopia	Optic tract/ radiation	Stroke, space-occupying lesions	
Homonymous hemianopia with macular sparing	Visual cortex	Stroke, space-occupying lesions	

37) Correct answer: D

Diffuse axonal injury occurs when shearing forces from trauma cause mechanical damage to axons, causing widescale damage to the brain itself. It is common in high speed motor vehicle accidents. The GCS is usually low and the CT scan may paradoxically be normal or show small punctate brain contusions or nothing dramatic. However, the injury to the brain is usually diffuse and therefore it is common to have severe neurological deficits from the injury. Treatment is supportive and prognosis is variable. All of the other injuries (extradural, subdural, hydrocephalus) would show up on a CT scan and are less likely to be caused by severe road traffic accidents.

Source: *Davidson's Principles and Practice of Surgery* (neurosurgery chapter)

38) Correct answer: E

This is an acute subdural haematoma. There is a crescent, concave, or banana-shaped hyperdensity (appears more bright than the surrounding brain tissue) that crosses suture lines. Hyperdensity can be from either acute blood or metal (blood being more likely in this case). This is consistent with an acute subdural. If the image was the same but the blood was hypodense (more black than the surrounding brain), it would be a chronic subdural haematoma. A system to interpreting CT head scans is crucial for exams, particularly OSCEs/clinical examination scenarios, and there aren't a lot of known systematic review methods like there are for ECGs and chest X-rays. The 'go from the outside to the inside approach' is recommended for junior doctors/clinical medical students to avoid missing important diagnoses:

Outside: circle around the bone, looking for any fractures

Then move inside the brain, circling the peripheries looking for any subdural or extradural haematomas

Then assess the grooves, looking for any signs of subarachnoid haemorrhage (see Paper 3, Question 40, Page 46)

Then assess the ventricles, looking for massive enlargement (hydrocephalus)

Then draw a line in the middle from the top down. If it is roughly equal, there is no midline shift; if It is not equal, there is midline shift, most likely as a result of a mass or bleed causing 'mass effect'.

A summary of how you would describe the above question scan is shown below (after, of course, describing the scan date, time, imaging method etc)

'There is no evidence of skull fractures. There is a right-sided crescent or concave-shaped hyperdensity that crosses suture lines with associated mass effect and midline shift. There is no evidence of subarachnoid haemorrhage or hydrocephalus, in keeping with an acute subdural haematoma. Urgent discussion with the on-call neurosurgical team is advised.'

39) Correct answer: B

The scan shows a large area of hypodensity (more black than surrounding brain tissue). This pattern is somewhat wedge-shaped/organised, and it covers a large territory of the brain. Causes of hypodensity on scans can either be infarction (dead tissue) or fluid. Infarcts often appear in such a pattern, and the massive territory affected indicates a large right-sided middle cerebral artery infarction. This patient is most likely to have suffered a significant stroke, which accounts for their neurological deficit on examination.

40) Correct answer: A

The correct diagnosis here is anterior cord syndrome. This is most common following a flexion injury, which would be caused by this gentleman flexing his neck from the bricks falling on him. The injury causes damage to the spinothalamic and corticospinal tracts, with subsequent loss or difficulty in sensing pain and temperature. The corticospinal tract is characteristically more affected in the lower areas, and this causes greater loss of power in the legs compared to the arms.

The opposite is central cord syndrome, which is caused by a hyperextension injury, and causes weakness of the arms but relative sparing of the LOWER limbs in contrast to anterior cord syndrome. Syringomyelia causes a classical 'cape distribution' sensory loss, with loss of pain and temperature and relative sparing of vibration and proprioception.

Spinal shock refers to a transient state of autonomic dysfunction that occurs after a severe spinal cord injury. As a result of damage to the autonomic pathways of the cord, you get marked hypotension and varying spinal cord dysfunction (flaccid paralysis, urinary retention, and faecal incontinence). Most patients have a prolonged recovery and need extensive rehabilitation afterwards.

Practice Paper 2 — Answers

1) Correct answer: D

Parkinson plus syndromes are often difficult to remember, so using some form of one sentence summary is really useful here. The correct answer is progressive supranuclear palsy, which is characterised by upward gaze palsy, having a fixed, 'surprised' look, and early falls that often lead to the patient using a wheelchair despite having normal power to avoid the falls (also known as 'wheelchair sign').

Multiple systems atrophy would fit with early falls, but you would need other forms of autonomic disturbance like gastroparesis, erectile dysfunction, demonstrated postural hypotension etc, as these are the predominant symptoms. Corticobasal degeneration can be remembered as having movement manifestations, such as 'alien limb' — where the patient describes having a limb (usually an arm) that they cannot control, is detached, or feels under the control of someone else — and myoclonus (electric shock-like jerks of a body part). Drug-induced Parkinson's is suggested if any patient is on medications that may reduce dopamine (the most common ones are antipsychotics which block the dopamine D2 receptor) and prokinetics like metoclopramide. The tremor is also commonly bilateral. For medical finals, knowing a simple sentence about the key features of each Parkinson plus syndrome should suffice.

2) Correct answer: C

This is classic multiple sclerosis. Thought to be caused by immune-mediated inflammatory plaques of demyelination from naive T helper cells crossing the blood-brain barrier, multiple sclerosis presents with neurological symptoms separated by time and space. This patient has two of these episodes, the first being optic neuritis (inflammation of the optic nerve), which causes a painful eye with blurred vision (visual acuity is often normal), and the second being difficulty differentiating colours such as red. Other episodes of neurological dysfunction include episodes of urinary incontinence and difficulty, as well as transient episodes of limb weakness and altered sensation. Other common but non-diagnostic features include Lhermitte's sign and Uhthoff's phenomenon (explained in Paper 3, Question 1, Page 33).

The most common subtype of multiple sclerosis is relapsing-remitting (over 70% of cases — marked by periods of relapse with symptoms followed by symptom-free intervals), but can also be primary-progressive, secondary-progressive, or progressive-relapsing. The clinical course of these symptoms is shown in the graphs below:

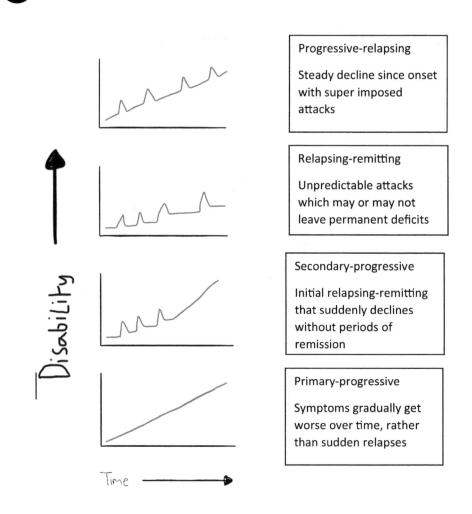

Progressive-relapsing

Steady decline since onset with super imposed attacks

Relapsing-remitting

Unpredictable attacks which may or may not leave permanent deficits

Secondary-progressive

Initial relapsing-remitting that suddenly declines without periods of remission

Primary-progressive

Symptoms gradually get worse over time, rather than sudden relapses

Disability

Time

Diagnosis is supported by MRI, which may show contrast-enhancing white matter lesions.

Treatment of an acute episode is with steroids (most commonly methylprednisolone), and for longer term treatment drugs such as natalizumab (monoclonal antibody), beta interferon, dimethyl fumarate and alemtuzumab are used. These all basically work on reducing the number or activity of the T cells or immune response thought to contribute to the disease. There is no cure for multiple sclerosis, and it is a high cause of morbidity to many.

3) Correct answer: A

The only medication known to improve prognosis in patients with motor neurone disease is riluzole, a glutamate receptor antagonist. This reduces the concentration of glutamate, an excess of which is thought to contribute towards motor neurone damage in the disease. The drug only improves survival by a 3–6 months, and this should be communicated to the patient. Steroids like prednisolone and dexamethasone have no effect on prognosis, tetrabenazine is a medication used for severe chorea in Huntington's, and natalizumab is a monoclonal antibody used in the treatment of refractory multiple sclerosis.

4) Correct answer: C

Huntington's disease is an autosomal dominant inherited trinucleotide repeat disorder and causes chorea, early dementia, and death in those affected. Being a trinucleotide repeat disorder, Huntington's exhibits the phenomenon of 'anticipation' — meaning subsequent generations are affected earlier and more severely. The chances of him passing his condition on to any child is 50%, as can be explained by the genetic cross below. People with autosomal dominant conditions are generally heterozygous (one normal copy and one bad copy) for the gene they carry, and with his wife not being affected she can be assumed to have two normal alleles:

		Mother (unaffected female)	
		h	h
Father (affected male)	H	Hh	Hh
	h	hh	hh

*H = huntington gene

The following are autosomal dominant neurological conditions: Huntington's, tuberous sclerosis, hereditary haemorrhagic telangiectasia, Charcot-Marie-Tooth disease, CADASIL.

The following are autosomal recessive neurological conditions: Tay-Sachs disease.

The following neurological disorders express genetic 'anticipation': Huntington's, Friedreich's ataxia, myotonic dystrophy.

5) Correct answer: B

This lady has had a psychogenic seizure, which is also called a non-epileptic attack disorder (NEAD). There are several features in her history that indicate this to be the case. First, the seizure lasted ten minutes. If this was an epileptic seizure, she would be in status epilepticus, a medical emergency. She also has her eyes shut, and many patients with NEAD will shut their eyes and resist an examiner from opening them during an episode. In most seizures, the eyes are open and the patient classically bites the SIDE of the tongue, but this lady had bitten the central part of it. Incontinence is variable and can occur in both NEADs and seizures, and in epileptic seizures the recovery time is often prolonged, with the person appearing 'groggy' for anywhere between 5 minutes and an hour afterwards. In NEAD, patients may recover quickly. Another key point is that seizures will often have the same pattern (such as limb jerking or tonic-clonic features), whereas NEAD may affect different limbs during different episodes. The key differences between epilepsy and NEAD are outlined in the table below:

Symptom	Epilepsy	NEAD/Psychogenic
Duration (minutes)	0.5–2 (unless in status)	Can be Longer than 2
Pelvic thrusting	Rare	Occasional
Eyes/mouth	Open	Closed
Side to side head movement	No	Yes
Tongue biting	Side	Anterior
Crying	Rare	More common
Talking	Rare	More common
Incontinence	Yes	Yes
Asymmetrical seizure pattern	No	Yes
Recovery	Slow	Fast

Conversion disorder occurs when a psychological event or strain of some sort is converted into a physical symptom, such as spontaneous leg weakness. It is most common in young adult females and often mimics neurological disorders such as a stroke and seizures. A classic feature is the so-called 'belle indifference', where a patient will not be stressed or concerned by their newfound deficit. Treatment is conservative and the patient should fully recover with psychological support.

Malingering is the feigning of an injury or problem for external gains, which are often obvious in the history. A wise clinician once told me, NEVER diagnose malingering! (always get someone else to do it for you due to the legal implications if you are wrong!!).

6) Correct answer: D

The patient is in status epilepticus, defined as continuous seizures lasting for more than 5 minutes, or repeated seizures between which consciousness is not fully recovered. His previous brain surgery is the most likely trigger for this. Status epilepticus is a medical emergency as it can cause brain damage from hypoxia and even death, and should be managed in a stepwise fashion (shown in the flow chart below). First, stabilise the airway in an A-E approach whilst calling for help. This includes, crucially, checking blood glucose to rule out hypoglycaemia. After this, the first treatment to give is intravenous lorazepam 4 mg, which can be repeated after 10 minutes if the patient is not responding. This is the first line treatment and can be given without delay in this patient because they have a cannula in situ. You should remember this drug and the dose as it will help you immensely both in exams and in real life as a doctor.

If this is unsuccessful, the next step is intravenous phenytoin (15–25 mg/kg), and at this point anaesthetic guidance should be sought. If this is again unsuccessful, you could then give phenobarbital (an anaesthetic agent) or consider intubation and ITU care.

If you are in the community such as a GP or have no intravenous access available, it is appropriate to manage status epilepticus with either rectal diazepam 10 mg or buccal (under

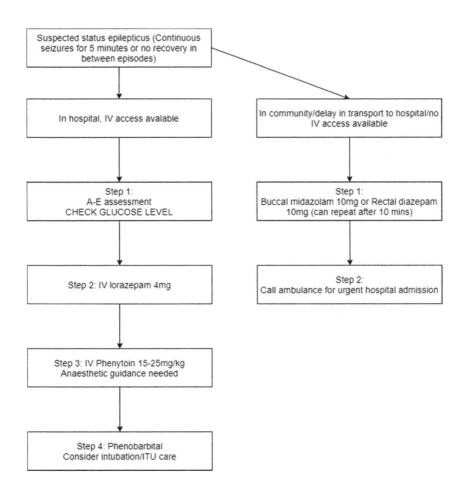

the tongue) midazolam 10 mg. These can be repeated after 10 minutes if no response is observed.

Status epilepticus management pathway.

7) Correct answer: C

This woman has classic migraine and, considering her symptoms, should be treated with prophylaxis. The first line treatment for prevention of migraine is propranolol. However, this is contraindicated due to her history of asthma. Second line treatment is topiramate, but this is also contraindicated as she is currently pregnant and topiramate is teratogenic. This should be mentioned to any woman of childbearing age who is started on it, and the importance of using contraception should be emphasised. Codeine is not effective for migraines, so amitriptyline should be offered. If all these treatments fail, more specialist treatments should be considered, such as acupuncture, botulinum toxin (botox) injections, and specialist neurology referral.

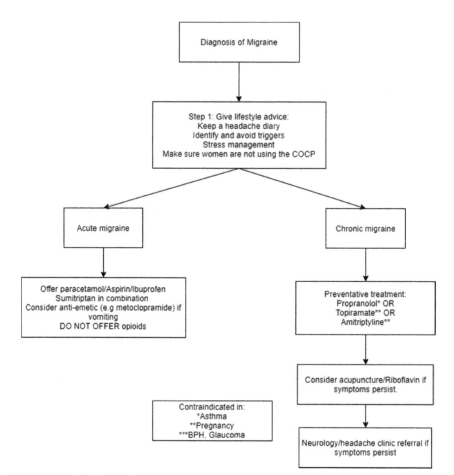

Source: NICE Guidelines for Migraine

8) Correct answer: D

This lady most likely has giant cell arteritis (GCA) and should be treated as such until indicated otherwise. As bloods have already been sent for ESR (an ESR over 50 makes the diagnosis likely), the appropriate next step is to start her on high-dose steroids like prednisolone (60–80 mg), which is effective for GCA and can lead to symptom resolution in a few days, along with a proton pump inhibitor to protect the stomach and possibly a bisphosphonate for bone protection if she is to be on it long term. Giving 15–20 mg is low dose and would be used for polymyalgia rheumatica only, and because a complication of untreated GCA is visual damage and blindness, she should be started on treatment immediately before any referrals are made.

GCA is a large vessel vasculitis often affecting the temporal arteries (it is often called temporal arteritis) and should be considered in any patient over the age of 50 presenting with new onset headache. The headache is classically brought on by touching the area near the temporal arteries, and actions like hair combing can exacerbate it. Patients may have other symptoms, with 15–20% having symptoms of polymyalgia rheumatica (weakness predominantly affecting the upper limbs) and jaw claudication (having pain or difficulty chewing and swallowing food). On examination, the temporal arteries may be tender or pulsatile. Diagnosis can be made using the American College of Rheumatology criteria, which considers symptoms, an ESR of over 50, and temporal artery biopsy in the diagnosis (although biopsy is often not conclusive as it can miss areas of inflammation).

Treatment is with long term (often 1–2 years of treatment) high-dose steroids (prednisolone), which often act very quickly, and support for the potential side effects of this (proton pump inhibitors, bisphosphonates) for gastric ulcer and osteoporosis prevention respectively.

9) Correct answer: A

This case is myaesthenia gravis, an immune-mediated disorder that leads to destruction of the post-synaptic nicotinic acetylcholine (ACh) receptor. This is important because ACh at synapses binds to the motor end plate, which causes muscles to contract. Damage to these channels reduces the effective ACh the body has for contraction, causing fatiguability, which is most common towards the end of the day, and can be demonstrated on examination as weakness that develops after a repetitive movement like making a fist. Patients may also get swallowing difficulty and eye problems, with diplopia being most common. Diagnosis is made based on clinical examination and edrophonium tests — this is the administration of a short-acting anticholinesterase inhibitor (AChi), which causes relief of symptoms. 10% of cases are associated with malignancy, the most common being a thymoma (tumour of the thymus), so investigating this with chest scanning should be considered. Treatment is with LONG- OR SHORT-acting AChi like pyridostigmine.

The opposite of myaesthenia gravis is Lambert-Eaton myaesthenic syndrome, whereby destruction of the presynaptic calcium channels of the motor end plate leads to a lack of calcium which causes the ACh release and subsequent muscle contraction. As a result, you get weakness that IMPROVES after repeated movements as calcium builds up to cause eventual ACh release. It is often a paraneoplastic syndrome (associated with malignancy), and 25% have malignancy with the syndrome, the most common cause being lung cancer.

10) Correct answer: C

In acute ischaemic stroke, depending on the time window that patients present in, they may be eligible for thrombolysis or thrombectomy. Thrombolysis involves intravenous administration of a tissue plasminogen activator (tPa), most commonly alteplase, which activates plasminogen to form plasmin, which then breaks down the clot in the brain that is causing the stroke. Thrombectomy is an interventional radiology procedure and involves removal of the clot manually by a catheter inserted into the patient's groin.

Thrombolysis is indicated within 4.5 hours of symptom onset and should be given intravenously by an experienced stroke physician and team only. The patient must not have any contraindications to this treatment, the main ones being uncertain time of onset

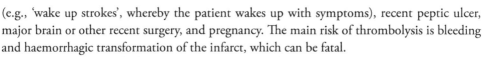

(e.g., 'wake up strokes', whereby the patient wakes up with symptoms), recent peptic ulcer, major brain or other recent surgery, and pregnancy. The main risk of thrombolysis is bleeding and haemorrhagic transformation of the infarct, which can be fatal.

Thrombectomy, which is an interventional radiology procedure whereby a catheter is inserted into the patient's groin to manually remove the clot causing the stroke, can be performed within 6 hours of symptom onset and has less risks than thrombolysis. Availability is an issue in many centres in the UK, such as being available only 9–5 Monday to Friday in some centres. In some circumstances, it can be used up to 24 hours of symptom onset, but these indications are rare and decided by specialists.

11) Correct answer: B

The Oxford-Bamford classification is used to classify stroke based on three clinical features: unilateral weakness and/or sensory disturbance affecting the arms or legs, homonymous hemianopia, and higher cortical disturbance such as Broca's or Wernicke's dysphasia. This patient has all three, and because the weakness is on the left-hand side, a stroke affecting the right-hand side of the brain caused it and thus it is called a right total anterior circulatory stroke (confusing, I know!). If a patient has 2 of the 3 (or just higher cortical dysfunction), it is called a partial anterior circulatory stroke, and if they have 1 of the 3, it is classed as a lacunar stroke. Typically examinable but easily learnable, you should definitely know the table below for med school finals:

Bamford stroke classification			
Total anterior circulatory stroke	Partial anterior circulatory stroke	Lacunar stroke	Posterior circulatory stroke
All three of: • Unilateral weakness • Homonymous hemianopia • Higher cerebral dysfunction (e.g., dysphasia)	Two of: • Unilateral weakness • Homonymous hemianopia • Higher cerebral dysfunction	One of: • Pure sensory stroke • Pure motor stroke • Sensorimotor stroke • Ataxic hemiparesis	One of: • Cranial nerve palsy and a contralateral motor/sensory deficit • Conjugate eye movements (e.g., gaze palsy) • Cerebellar dysfunction (e.g., ataxia, nystagmus, vertigo) • Isolated homonymous hemianopia or cortical blindness

12) Correct answer: B

This patient has presented with signs of personality change, most markedly loss of inhibition (becoming more aggressive and rude, gambling), and inability to function. This is generally referred to as the 'dysexecutive syndrome' and occurs in lesions or damage to the frontal lobe of the brain, where the prefrontal cortex is responsible for higher executive functioning. Parietal lobe lesions would present with sensation change, temporal lobe lesions would present with problems with memory, hearing, and occasionally speech if Wernicke's area is affected, and there are no visual changes reported in the case which rules out an occipital lesion. The train track injury is the most likely cause of his symptoms, and the case closely resembles that of Phineas Gage, a respectful man who became much more aggressive and disinhibited with marked personality change after a railing pipe impaled his frontal lobe.

13) Correct answer: C

Classic Alzheimer's disease. Gradual decline in memory, reduction in higher functions (like crossword puzzles), and forgetfulness that is worse at night (this is often seen in dementia) all point towards a diagnosis of Alzheimer's. A MOCA score of less than 23 is considered abnormal, so this patient's score of 17 suggests significant cognitive impairment. Mild cognitive impairment would present with a much milder memory decline and not cause much disruption to functional life like how it is in this case; vascular dementia would be suggested if the patient had a vascular history like ischaemic heart disease or repeated strokes, and a classic 'stepwise progression' of cognitive deficit would be present. Frontotemporal dementia would usually present in a relatively younger patient (aged 50s–60s) and marked personality change would be a prominent feature. In Alzheimer's, patients often make a good attempt at responding to questions, whereas someone with depressive pseudodementia may simply reply 'I don't know' to questions asked and be worried about having dementia themselves, as well as having other symptoms of depression.

Alzheimer's disease is the most common form of dementia, causes a gradual decline in memory and higher cognitive functioning, and is due to the build-up of amyloid and tau protein deposits in the brain, causing atrophy. Risk factors include increased age, cardiovascular disease, trisomy 21 (so-called because the amyloid precursor protein is located on chromosome 21), and low educational status. Patients may report getting lost frequently in places that were previously familiar, 'leaving the hobs turned on', and not recognising people they know. Short-term memory is affected first. There is no cure and the only treatments available are acetylcholinesterase inhibitors like donepezil, galantamine, and rivastigmine for mild to moderate dementia (increasing ACh is thought to reduce rate of memory decline) and memantine (a glutamate receptor antagonist) for moderate to severe dementia.

14) Correct answer: D

This is Guillain-Barré syndrome, also known as acute inflammatory demyelinating polyradiculopathy. It usually appears 1–3 weeks after a respiratory or gastrointestinal infection, and the most common causative organism is *Campylobacter jejuni*. It presents with distal sensory loss and patchy weakness, with symptoms ascending up the body over a few days, as well as loss of tendon reflexes (hence why it is called ascending areflexic paralysis). In patients with cranial nerve or bulbar involvement, the big problem is intercostal and diaphragmatic weakness causing respiratory failure, and vital capacity must be monitored to decide if the patient needs ventilation.

Diagnosis is usually clinical, supported by nerve conduction studies that show reduced nerve conduction speed, and lumbar puncture may show raised cerebrospinal fluid protein and a normal cell count or mild lymphocytosis.

Patients need careful monitoring of respiratory and cardiac function, and in severe cases can be treated with intravenous immunoglobulin and occasionally plasmapheresis. Most patients recover, but roughly 5% die due to complications.

Source: Crash Course Neurology, 5th Edition (2018).

15) Correct answer: D

The medical research council's (MRC) power scale is commonly examined even in final year OSCEs, so it is worth knowing given the significant chance that it will appear. Any neurological exam should consist of sensation, motor, cerebellar, and cranial nerve examinations. When making motor assessments, the MRC grades of power are used and are shown below. This patient has movement that is possible with gravity eliminated (by putting the arm and legs flat on the examination couch) and would therefore classify as grade 2.

MRC Grade	Description
0	No movement
1	Flicker of contraction
2	Active movement possible if gravity eliminated
3	Active movement against gravity but not resistance
4	Active movement against gravity and resistance but not full power
5	Normal power

16) Correct answer: B

This patient has a Holmes-Adie pupil, a benign finding of a dilated pupil which does not react to light but slowly reacts to accommodation. The finding may also be accompanied by generalised hyporeflexia (again a benign finding) indicating Holmes-Adie syndrome. It does not require investigation or treatment.

A relative afferent pupillary defect is pupillary dilation that occurs when light is moved from the contralateral eye to the affected eye (it should normally constrict). It is a sign of retinal or optic disc disease, and the most common causes are optic neuritis in young people and retinal disease in the elderly.

An Argyll Robertson pupil is a miotic (small) pupil that does not constrict to light but constricts to accommodation, and it is associated with tertiary syphilis. Both the absence of syphilis in the history and the dilated pupil make this diagnosis unlikely in this case.

A third cranial nerve palsy would present with limited eye movements, with the pupil in a 'down and out' pattern, and ptosis which are not present here.

17) Correct answer: E

The patient is describing myoclonus. Terms to describe abnormal movements are easily remembered with one sentence summaries:

Myoclonus is sudden and brief shock-like contractions described as jerking or startling.

Dystonia is involuntary muscle contraction causing twisting or repetitive movements or abnormal postures.

Tremors are involuntary rhythmic movements of a limb or body part which is shaking, jerking, or twitching in nature.

Chorea are brief and irregular flowing movements, often described as 'dance-like'.

Athetosis refers to slow, writhing, non-purposeful, and often flowing movements.

Tardive dyskinesia refers to irregular non-purposeful movements such as lip smacking.

Akathisia refers to motor restlessness.

Hemiballismus involves involuntary unilateral large-amplitude flinging movements.

Movement type	Description	Seen in
Myoclonus	Sudden, brief shock-like contractions described as jerking or startling	Benign myoclonus, uraemia, medications (lithium)
Dystonia	Involuntary muscle contraction causing twisting or repetitive movements or abnormal postures	Primary dystonia Secondary: stroke
Tremor	Involuntary rhythmic movement of a limb or body part which is shaking, jerking, or twitching in nature	Parkinson's Benign essential tremor Medications (beta 2 agonists)
Chorea	Brief irregular, flowing movements (often described as 'dance-like')	Huntington's
Athetosis	Slow, writhing, non-purposeful and often flowing movements	Stroke, basal ganglia disorders
Tardive Dyskinesia	Irregular non-purposeful movements such as lip smacking	Prolonged antipsychotic use
Akathisia	Motor restlessness	Antipsychotic use
Hemiballismus	Involuntary unilateral large-amplitude flinging movements	Ischaemic stroke

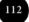

18) Correct answer: C

This young boy has all the cutaneous features of neurofibromatosis type 1 (NF1). NF1 is an autosomal dominant inherited condition and it is the most common type (1 in 2500 people). Patients are at increased risk of malignancies (most commonly optic nerve gliomas, neurofibroma, and glioma) as well as haematological cancers like leukaemia and neuroblastoma. The characteristic skin features are café au lait spots (light brown macules), axillary freckling, and neurofibromas, all of which this patient has.

Neurofibromatosis type 2 (NF2) is less common (1 in 50,000), the skin manifestations are not usually present, and patients have the pathognomonic feature of bilateral vestibular schwannomas (acoustic neuromas), or tumours of the Schwann cells that line the vestibular nerve. They are also at risk of meningioma and cataracts.

Tuberous sclerosis is explained separately in Paper 3, Question 18, Page 38.

Sturge-Weber syndrome is a congenital neurocutaneous syndrome, with hallmark features of a facial port wine stain, abnormally fragile blood vessels on the brain surface, and ocular problems (most commonly glaucoma). This is very rarely asked in finals, so don't bother learning it!

19) Correct answer: C

The vomiting centre is located in the medulla, a part of the brainstem, and is responsible for controlling vomiting. It contains histamine (H1) and acetylcholine receptors, and drugs that act on these to prevent vomiting include cyclizine.

The postrema area, located at the floor of the fourth ventricle in the brain, is where the chemoreceptor trigger zone is located. This area is responsible for sending signals linked to vomiting to the vomiting centre and contains serotonin (5HT3) and dopamine (D2) receptors. Blocking these receptors with drugs like ondansetron (a 5HT3 antagonist) and prochlorperazine (a D2 antagonist) can control vomiting.

20) Correct answer: B

This case describes a textbook acute Extradural haematoma. Caused by rupture of the middle meningeal artery (MMA) often as a result of trauma over a weakened part of the skull (pterion), it causes a characteristic 'lucid interval' of apparent recovery followed by a drop in consciousness level. CT head scan will show a convex, lens shaped hyperdensity (whiteness) of acute blood which generally does not cross suture lines, and there may be an associated skull fracture. Urgent Neurosurgical referral is advised for guidance and possible transfer and surgery.

Acute subdural haematoma is explained in paper 1, question 29, page 10.

Post-concussion syndrome would present weeks to months after the injury and is characterised by mild cognitive difficulties, often accompanied by personality change. Management is conservative and outcomes are favourable.

Malignant MCA syndrome is explained in Paper 3, question 6, page 34.

21) Correct answer: D

This mass is most likely to be a Meningioma, an often benign tumour of the meninges that line the brain. They are frequently discovered in asymptomatic patients (like this one), and appear as spherical masses often located separately to the brain, do not invade it and may be calcified. There also may be surrounding hyperostosis (extra bone) due to bone invasion.

Management is by active observation with MRI scans, and most can be surgically removed without complication if the patient becomes symptomatic (most commonly seizures).

Glioblastoma (GB) is less likely in this patient because it often presents with the patient being symptomatic, often with a subacute decline in neurological function- there is also brain invasion, and the tumour may appear irregular, vascular or necrotic on scans (Paper 3, Question 19, page 38).

Medulloblastoma is less likely given the patients age (it most commonly affects children in the first decade of life), there is no mention to suggest previous brain surgery ruling out gliosis (fancy term for brain scarring) and astrocytoma is more common in children, and would be located in the brain itself.

22) Correct answer: D

There is only one real answer here: this is the textbook example of a subarachnoid haemorrhage. The characteristic features are thunderclap headache (reaches maximum intensity within 5 minutes of onset) or the 'worst ever headache', which is often described as being hit over the head with something (often a bat of some sort), and it is often triggered by exertion (e.g., exercise, sexual intercourse). There is also neck stiffness as the blood in the subarachnoid space can cause meningeal irritation.

The most common cause of a subarachnoid haemorrhage is actually trauma, but for exam purposes it is also good to be aware that they can be caused by the rupture of saccular (or 'berry') aneurysms, and risk factors include autosomal dominant polycystic disease and hypertension. All patients will need to be admitted to hospital with regular neurological observations and a CT head scan (which can identify up to 95% of subarachnoid haemorrhages within 24 hrs). If this is negative, perform a lumbar puncture at 12 hrs for bilirubin (a yellow appearance that resembles blood breakdown products indicates a subarachnoid haemorrhage).

An aneurysm may need coiling or clipping if it is found to be the cause, and subarachnoid haemorrhage carries a high mortality rate (50% die before reaching the hospital). Complications of subarachnoid haemorrhage are discussed in Paper 3, Question 25, Page 40.

23) Correct answer: A

The most likely diagnosis here is degenerative cervical myelopathy (DCM). Motor neurone disease is less likely as there are only upper motor neuron signs specifically on examination, while primary lateral sclerosis is just a subtype of motor neurone disease where the corticospinal tract is primarily affected. He only has symptoms affecting the hands which rules out lumbar radiculopathy, and his profile does not fit that of the typical multiple sclerosis patient (young female, eye problems etc).

DCM is a common neurodegenerative condition that often occurs due to spinal cord compression at the level of the cervical spine, and it is linked to cervical spondylosis. Patients present with weakness and difficulty using both arms and hands due to compression of the cervical spinal cord, and symptoms are usually progressive over many months. On examination, there may be loss of reflexes and flaccid weakness at the level of the lesion, but spasticity and increased reflexes below it. One of the pathological reflexes may be present: Babinski's sign, clonus, or Hoffman's sign may be positive (flicking the middle finger causes reflex contractions of the thumb and index finger). Patients with suspected DCM should undergo an MRI scan of the cervical spine and be referred to neurological or spine surgery services for consideration of surgical decompression, which may relieve the pressure on the cord and subsequent symptoms. The disease is progressive and surgery only stops progression, often without benefit to symptoms.

Myelopathy.org is a good website for further information on the condition!

24) Correct answer: C

The correct answer is cauda equina syndrome. A lumbar disc prolapse would not usually present with urinary and bowel incontinence, and the pain may be neuropathic in nature (shooting down the leg) as well as having a dermatomal pattern. She has no systemic features to suggest malignancy, and an osteoporotic fracture would present with less severe weakness with more prominent back pain and possible loss of height.

The patient has all the key features of cauda equina: back pain, altered perianal sensation ('saddle' anaesthesia), and sphincter dysfunction (urinary and/or bowel retention and incontinence). She needs an urgent MRI of the lumbosacral spine with potential urgent neurosurgical referral for emergency decompressive surgery as she is fit and well.

Cauda equina syndrome is a medical emergency and can cause irreversible damage to sphincter function, leading to long-term bladder and bowel incontinence as well as neurological deficits. It is most often caused by herniation of a lumbar disc into the cauda equina (nerve roots that continue after the spinal cord ends), leading to compression and damage to the lower sacral nerves (S2–S4) and subsequently sensory, motor, and autonomic dysfunction as described above. It is more common in the elderly, but can affect any age group. The key features are bowel and/or bladder dysfunction, back pain, bilateral sciatica, leg weakness, and/or sensory dysfunction, and examination may reveal perianal 'saddle' anaesthesia.

Cauda equina is a significant cause of medical negligence claims and should never be missed. Patients need an urgent MRI of the whole spine to rule this out (usually within 12 hours).

Acute onset bladder and/or bowel dysfunction with perianal 'saddle' anaesthesia is cauda equina syndrome until proven otherwise, and urgent spinal MRI is essential to rule this out in all patients. Management is with urgent surgical decompression, preferably within 24 hours of symptom onset (NICE).

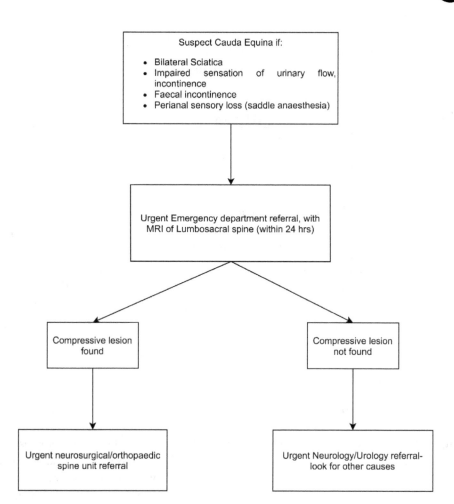

25) Correct answer: D

This patient has suffered uncal (transtentorial) herniation as a result of progression of his glioblastoma, producing mass effect and raising the intracranial pressure. The signs specific to uncal herniation are the dilated pupil on one side (often the ipsilateral side to the tumour) due to midbrain compression, as well as contralateral hemiparesis due to compression of the corticospinal tracts. A new onset stroke could be possible given the weakness, but with the pupil signs is less likely, and the patient has a brain tumour already which points more to herniation. Subfalcine herniation is usually less serious and the patient may not be gravely ill, and the breathing pattern is regular. In tonsillar herniation, the breathing centres are compressed, meaning that they may be irregular or the patient will be close to death. The main types of herniation are summarised in the table below:

Brain herniation occurs because the brain is effectively closed in a box (the skull). Too much pressure inside (from mostly tumours, bleeds, and trauma) can cause structures to move and press on others. The pressure on vital brain structures is what causes herniation and should be suspected in any patient with a traumatic brain injury. A known malignancy or bleed that suddenly deteriorates is life threatening and needs urgent senior review.

Type of herniation	Clinical features	Structures affected
Subfalcine	Most common herniation pattern Less severe than uncal and tonsillar headache, nausea and vomiting, altered mental status	Falx cerebri
Transtentorial (uncal)	Ipsilateral dilated pupil Contralateral hemiparesis Rarely ipsilateral hemiparesis due to Kernohan phenomenon	Medial temporal lobe
Tonsillar	Altered respiratory and cardiac function Most cases death	Cerebellar tonsils (arrow) — foramen magnum = brainstem compressed
All types	Can cause Cushing's triad: hypertension, bradycardia, irregular respiration	

26) Correct answer: B

This is characteristic cavernous sinus thrombosis. Painful ophthalmoplegia, proptosis, and chemosis after a recent facial or sinus infection are highly indicative. Pituitary apoplexy may cause similar presenting symptoms but is less likely, because while it can cause cavernous sinus thrombosis, she does not have a pituitary tumour, and it is often an acute presentation. A posterior communicating artery aneurysm presents with painful third cranial nerve palsy (this patient also has the fifth cranial nerve affected as evidenced by the facial numbness).

The cavernous sinus is a pair of blood-filled spaces on either side of the pituitary gland and contains critical structures that pass through it (see table).

Cranial nerves	Oculomotor (third cranial nerve) Trochlear (fourth cranial nerve) V1 and V2 branches of trigeminal (fifth cranial nerve) Abducens (sixth cranial nerve)
Arteries	Internal carotid artery

Cavernous sinus thrombosis can cause compression of all of these structures and characteristically affects them. The causes are often due to infection (e.g., facial infection, sinusitis) spreading to the cavernous sinus, malignancy with spread to the sinus, or idiopathic factors. Classical features are painful ophthalmoplegia (from compression of the cranial nerves that move the eyes), chemosis (periorbital tissue oedema), and eyeball protrusion (proptosis). You may also get loss of facial sensation due to trigeminal nerve compression and papilloedema from ophthalmic vein dilatation. Complications include visual loss and intracranial spread of the original infection or malignancy.

Management is dependent on the cause: those linked to infections should be managed with antibiotics, idiopathic causes should be managed with anticoagulants, and suspected malignancy should be referred to specialists depending on the primary site.

Pituitary apoplexy is an acute haemorrhage into the pituitary gland, usually associated with a pituitary tumour (Paper 5, Question 14, page 67) with subsequent infarction into the pituitary gland. It can cause acute cavernous sinus syndrome and requires emergency neurosurgical review.

27) Correct answer: C

This gentleman most likely has a progressive brain tumour given the suspicious mass and prominent oedema, and dexamethasone is commonly used to manage peritumoral oedema, which can help to reduce compression of vital neurological structures and minimize associated symptoms. Mannitol could be suitable as it is an osmotic diuretic used to acutely reduce raised intracranial pressure, but dexamethasone is a better option in the presence of a known tumour. There is no indication for morphine sulphate, and acetazolamide is used in acute angle closure glaucoma to reduce intraocular pressure, and can also be used for the treatment of idiopathic intracranial hypertension. Nimodipine is a calcium channel blocker that is used to reduce vasospasm in cases of subarachnoid haemorrhage.

28) Correct answer: C

This gentleman unfortunately has the symptoms of tertiary syphilis, and the maculopapular rash he describes from 20 years ago is likely a manifestation of secondary syphilis. He has several features of neurosyphilis to boot — Argyll Robertson pupils, signs of tabes dorsalis (degeneration of the dorsal columns creating impaired proprioception and vibration), stroke at a young age (most likely another manifestation of tertiary syphilis), and general paresis (dementia and motor symptoms such as myoclonus). Creutzfeldt-Jakob disease is possible in this patient, but is less likely given the prolonged history of neurovascular events and syphilis symptoms proceeding from it (there would be a rapid decline). Bipolar disorder would not cause such neurological manifestations and this is part of general paresis. Frontotemporal dementia would also present with less motor manifestations and more prominent personality change with memory loss.

Tertiary syphilis is a rare manifestation of untreated syphilis infection (only 7% cases of untreated syphilis) and thus is rare. They classically occur between 10 and 20 years after the initial infection and can manifest in several ways:

Symptom	Time after primary infection	Details
Meningovascular syphilis	5–10 years	Meningitis stroke **(in a young person)**
Argyll Robertson pupils	10–20 years	Pupils do not react to light but slowly to accommodation, small pupils
General paresis	15–20 years	Dementia, manic behaviour, paralysis, myoclonus
Tabes dorsalis	15–10 years	Lightning pains, loss of joint proprioception and vibration (falls, Charcot joint)

Other manifestations include spinal and optic atrophy. Treatment is with benzylpenicillin injections, but in tertiary syphilis it is often not enough.

29) Correct answer: C

This young patient has no concerning features of head injury that would merit a CT scan as he is alert, fully orientated, does not have a neurological deficit, and has no signs of a basal skull fracture (see Paper 1, Question 5, Page 2). Therefore, apart from active neurological observations to make sure that there is no evolving head injury like an expanding bleed or extradural injury, no CT scan is required. He also has no neck stiffness or concerns of a cervical spine fracture, so an X-ray of the cervical spine is not indicated.

30) Correct answer: C

Spinal cord levels of reflexes are commonly tested in OSCE scenarios at every level of medical school (even up to finals on occasion), so the basic ones (e.g., dermatomes) should be memorised:

Reflex	Spinal cord level
Biceps	C5–C6
Supinator	C6
Triceps	C7–C8
Patellar (knee)	L2–L4
Ankle	S1–S2
Babinski	S1

31) Correct answer: B

Baclofen is an antispasticity agent that is used as adjunct therapy in patients with multiple sclerosis, whereby spasticity causes pain or interruption of daily life. Pyridostigmine is a short-acting acetylcholinesterase inhibitor that inhibits the enzyme that breaks down acetylcholine, so it is used for myaesthenia gravis. Diazepam can be used as medication to reduce spasticity, but not as first line treatment due to its considerable side effect profile (e.g., addiction, drowsiness). Aspirin is not used for spasticity, and neither is propranolol.

32) Correct answer: A

This patient has suffered from a lumbar disc protrusion (also called disc prolapse/herniation). This is where the intervertebral disc 'slips', compressing the nerve roots of the spinal cord and producing symptoms. There is classically low back pain and sciatica (pain radiation from the back to the buttock and leg). Onset is typically acute and follows a lifting, bending, or minor injury, but may also be spontaneous. On examination, straight leg raise may be limited, and there is loss of reflex such as ankle jerks as well as weakness of plantar flexion or great toe extension. Sensory loss over the L4-S1 dermatomes may also be present, like in this case. It can be diagnosed with a spine MRI, which will show the protrusion.

Management of sciatica and lumbar disc protrusion is conservative, as most cases resolve within 12 weeks with rest and analgesia. Surgery is only indicated when a significant disc protrusion is persistent, symptomatic, or severe and corticosteroid joint injections have not been effective.

Source: Kumar and Clark's Clinical Medicine, 10th Edition (2020).

33) Correct answer: C

This patient is suffering from an acute stress reaction. This occurs in response to exceptional physical and/or psychological stress. While severe, such a reaction usually subsides within days. The stress is often an overwhelming traumatic experience, such as an accident, physical or sexual assault, or death. Acute stress reaction often involves feeling 'dazed' or numb, with strange neurological symptoms such as reported loss of vision but no visible defects on examination. Most cases resolve within a month. No treatments beyond reassurance and support are normally necessary.

Source: Goldman-Cecil Medicine, 26th Edition (2020).

34) Correct answer: B

Multiple sclerosis is considered to have four clinical patterns:

Relapsing-remitting: the most common type (85% of patients with multiple sclerosis), involving relapses of unpredictable clinical deterioration followed by periods of remission, with less recovery as disease goes on.

Primary-progressive: 10–15% of patients with multiple sclerosis, more common in men, progressive neurological disability from symptom onset, no remissions.

Secondary-progressive: 40–50% of patients with relapsing-remitting multiple sclerosis develop this after 10–15 years; no more relapses, only progressive neurological symptoms and decline.

Progressive-relapsing: Least common pattern (5–10%) — progressive disease from onset with exacerbations.

*Source: Eureka! Neurology and Neurosurgery (2016).

35) Correct answer: C

This is a partial seizure (abnormal seizure activity is restricted to one part of the brain) because of the lack of generalised symptoms like tonic-clonic movements of arms and legs. The temporal lobe is known to produce 'odd' seizure symptoms such as feelings of familiarity (déjà vu) and non-familiarity (jamais vu), gustatory (taste), olfactory (smell), and complex motor phenomena, as well as a 'rising epigastric sensation'. These are often called 'automatisms' and consist of things like lip smacking and chewing.

Any of these symptoms should prompt you to suspect the temporal lobe as the region affected by the seizure. The frontal lobe is characterised by motor dysfunction, expressive speech difficulty, and behaviour changes. Parietal lobe seizures have abnormal sensations or sensory dysfunction and possible motor symptoms due to involvement of the frontal lobe, while occipital lobe seizures have visual symptoms such as flashing lights.

36) Correct answer: A

Verapamil (calcium channel blocker) is the first line treatment for the prevention of cluster headache. Propranolol is the first line treatment for migraine prevention. Lithium is a second line agent for prevention of cluster headache and should only be initiated by a specialist. Topiramate is also used for migraine, and primidone is used for the management of benign essential tremor.

For cluster headache explanations, see Paper 1, Question 16, Page 6.

37) Correct answer: D

The Recognition of Stroke in The Emergency Room score is used to assess the possibility of stroke in the emergency department and looks at symptoms and signs that more or less suggestive of stroke. This includes asymmetric facial, arm or leg weakness, speech disturbance, and visual field defects, with points lost for loss of consciousness or seizure activity. A score of more than 0 indicates that a stroke is possible and should be treated as such. It is better than the FAST score (face, arms, speech time) because FAST does not include posterior circulation stroke symptoms (e.g., vertigo, diplopia, ataxia) or stroke mimics and is often used by ambulance crews but not emergency doctors.

The National Institute of Health Stroke Scale is a more detailed stroke score used by specialist stroke physicians to evaluate the extent of a stroke, including motor, speech, language, vision, and interpretation tests, and is scored out of 42 points.

The ABCD^2 score is used in transient ischaemic attack management to assess the risk of an imminent future stroke and is scored as follows:

Feature	Score
Age: >60 yrs	1
Blood pressure	
>140/90 or currently undergoing treatment for hypertension	1
Clinical features	
Unilateral weakness	2
Speech disturbance	1
Any other symptoms	0
Duration of symptoms	
0–10 minutes	0
10–59 minutes	1
>59 minutes	2
Diabetes	
Yes	1
No	0

A score of 4 or over is bad and indicates a 7-day stroke risk of 6–11%, and those with a score of 2 or more should be referred to a stroke specialist for assessment, investigations, and possible preventative treatment, usually with an antiplatelet such as clopidogrel (now first line, although ticagrelor is becoming increasingly used), aspirin, or dipyridamole/ticagrelor.

38) Correct answer: C

This image displays an acute extradural haematoma. As stated in Paper 1, there is an underlying temporal bone fracture and a brightness on the scan (hyperdensity) that does not cross suture lines, and the haematoma is convex or lens-shaped in nature. This suggests the presence of acute blood and, in the context of the image, an extradural haematoma is the most likely diagnosis, with a good differential being an acute subdural haematoma. This patient will almost certainly require urgent neurosurgical management, such as evacuation of the haematoma.

39) Correct answer: D

This image shows a cerebral abscess. This is most likely as it has a classical well-defined 'rim' shape, coupled with the patient's history (fever, headaches and weakness is the triad for cerebral abscess, IVDU also contributes here). A meningioma would not have the rim and would be towards the edge of the brain (at least for exam purposes!). A glioblastoma would be large, irregular, and less spherical, there will be prominent oedema, and it will just look horrible on a scan. Finally, a colloid cyst would be smaller, fluid-filled entirely, and located in between the ventricles instead of the brain parenchyma itself.

40) Correct answer: A

This patient has classic delirium, which is likely linked to her recent surgery. Normally, the standard medical treatment for acute delirium is haloperidol, a dopamine D2 receptor antagonist. However, this patient has Lewy body dementia, so giving haloperidol in these patients can exacerbate Parkinsonian symptoms and cause clinical decline, even leading to death. NEVER prescribe antipsychotics of any kind in patients with Parkinson's disease or Lewy body dementia! A benzodiazepine (preferably a short-acting one) is the next best treatment here, so lorazepam fits the bill. Chlorpromazine is an antipsychotic that would worsen symptoms, while L-dopa would not help the delirium and acute agitation.

Practice Paper 3 — Answers

1) Correct answer: C

This patient is describing the Uhthoff phenomenon — the transient worsening of multiple sclerosis symptoms after an increase in body temperature — usually after exercise, fever, or being in a sauna or hot tub. This may manifest as multiple sclerosis symptoms that worsen with the aforementioned activities, and they are usually transient.

Lhermitte's sign describes electric shock-like pains in the hands and legs produced by neck flexion, which is also seen in multiple sclerosis. Hoover's relates to functional disorders. Internuclear ophthalmoplegia is a complex eye pattern seen in multiple sclerosis or stroke, in which the affected eye cannot adduct, along with nystagmus of the contralateral abducting eye. Brudzinski's sign describes knee and hip flexion on neck flexion and is seen in meningeal irritation or meningitis.

2) Correct answer: E

This patient is in status epilepticus as his seizure has now lasted more than 5 minutes, and an ambulance is at least half an hour away. As it is a medical emergency and waiting for an ambulance is not plausible, he needs urgent medical treatment. In this situation, it is clear that he has difficult intravenous access, and trying to gain access would only delay vital treatment. So although intravenous lorazepam is the first line treatment usually in status epilepticus in a hospital or healthcare setting, with poor intravenous access you should use buccal midazolam 10 mg or rectal diazepam 10–20 mg. This will mean that the patient can receive rapid treatment before the ambulance arrives. A glucose reading is normal, so he does not need glucagon, and there are no signs of anaphylaxis, so he does not need adrenaline. For an explanation of status epilepticus, see Paper 2, Question 6, Page 19.

3) Correct answer: B

This is a very concerning presentation, and a brain tumour or space-occupying lesion should be excluded with an urgent MRI or CT scan (within 2 weeks) depending on availability and her clinical status. This headache has almost all the features of raised intracranial pressure — it is often worse in the mornings and worse on lying flat, and there may be nausea, vomiting, and double vision. This can be due to tumour oedema or compression/stimulation of key structures like the vomiting centre or chemoreceptor trigger zone, which induce vomiting. The presentation is also progressively worsening which is concerning.

She has no weakness listed which rules out hemiplegic migraine, and she has no vertigo which rules out benign paroxysmal positional vertigo. Tension headache would present with 'band-like' bilateral headache and be less severe, and she lacks the classic features of Horner's syndrome (ptosis, miosis, enophthalmos, facial anhidrosis).

4) Correct answer: E

Idiopathic intracranial hypertension (IIH) has been explained in Paper 1, Question 4, Page 4. With IIH, the most effective proven treatment is weight loss of between 10–20% of body weight. The reasons for this are unclear, but IIH occurs most commonly in young, overweight females, some with polycystic ovary syndrome, so weight loss is recommended and is effective at alleviating symptoms. If this is not possible or the patient presents acutely with visual changes and/or papilloedema (as visual loss is the most dangerous complication of IIH), medication with acetazolamide (also used for acute glaucoma) can be attempted. More definitive options for refractory cases include a venoplasty (expansion of one of the major cerebral veins to improve venous outflow) or a shunt to divert cerebrospinal fluid and reduce intracranial pressure, but these are last resort therapies.

5) Correct answer: A

Sudden onset of dizziness and vertigo in any elderly patient or one with vascular risk factors? Think posterior circulatory stroke. This rarely presents with the usual stroke features (e.g., weakness, speech problems) and actually presents with sudden onset dizziness, vertigo, syncope, and sometimes diplopia.

   This patient needs to be considered for thrombolysis if it is within the time criteria, so an emergency CT head scan and urgent stroke team referral is the next step.

   Benign paroxysmal positional vertigo would be worsened by Dix-Hallpike's manoeuvre and would be resolved by Epley's, which involves holding the head over a bed and rotating it in different directions.

   Vestibular migraine would present with vertigo, dizziness, or balance disturbance with migraine-like features. The Meniere's triad of dizziness, vertigo, tinnitus, and sensorineural hearing loss is not present.

6) Correct answer: D

This patient has malignant middle cerebral artery (MCA) syndrome, a medical emergency that can cause raised intracranial pressure, brain shift, and subsequent coning (herniation of the brain with subsequent pressure on the breathing centres, leading to death). Malignant MCA syndrome occurs in large MCA infarcts where the area of infarct occupies more than 50% of the MCA territory on scanning. Subsequent cytotoxic oedema from dead tissue can cause significant brain swelling, which can lead to reduced consciousness and death if not treated. The treatment is with mannitol to reduce the intracranial pressure followed by urgent neurosurgery (if the patient is well enough) in the form of a decompressive craniectomy (literally removing part of the cranium, allowing the brain to expand outwards to relieve the pressure). Prognosis is poor but some patients do make a full recovery. The stroke team will most likely be managing the patient and should also be informed.

7) Correct answer: C

Firstly, this doctor is being mean expecting this diagnosis from a medical student. Nevertheless, third cranial nerve palsy with contralateral hemiplegia or hemiparesis is characteristic of Weber's syndrome. It is caused by midbrain infarction (most commonly a stroke), and that's all I would expect you to know for finals. Keep it simple.

Claude syndrome is the opposite and can be remembered by the mnemonic 'Weak Weber, Clumsy Claude', with a third cranial nerve palsy accompanied by ataxia.

Gerstmann's syndrome is finger agnosia, acalculia, agraphia, and confusion between the right- and left-hand sides, and is caused by a lesion or damage to the angular gyrus in the brain.

Wallenberg syndrome, also known as lateral medullary syndrome, is loss of pain sensation on one side of the face ipsilateral to the lesion, with loss of pain and temperature on the other side of the body with minimal to no weakness. You may also get an ipsilateral Horner's syndrome, vertigo, ataxia, and nystagmus. It is caused by a stroke infarction of the posterior inferior cerebellar artery more specifically.

Millard-Gubler syndrome is ipsilateral sixth and seventh cranial nerve palsy with contralateral hemiplegia.

Disclaimer: in-depth knowledge is not required for these topics for finals, so learning a sentence about them is more than enough.

8) Correct answer: C

This is textbook Lewy body dementia — visual hallucinations, fluctuating cognition, Parkinsonism, and sleep disturbances define the condition. It is due to Lewy body deposition and build-up of alpha synuclein, a toxic particle, and presents with the above listed symptoms. Management is controversial because traditional dementia therapies like acetylcholinesterase inhibitors cannot be administered as they may make the patient worse, so few effective treatments are available.

The other types of dementia are explained in Paper 2, Question 13, Page 21.

9) Correct answer: C

This patient most likely has encephalitis and should be managed urgently with intravenous acyclovir (antiviral treatment) and senior advice. The history is not convincing for meningitis as there is no prominent neck stiffness, headache, or photophobia, while seizures, confusion, and fever lasting over a week is more characteristic of encephalitis. There is no evidence to suggest that he is septic, so sepsis six is not the best answer, and intramascular (NOT intravenous) benzylpenicillin should be given if you suspect meningitis to be in the community.

Encephalitis is inflammation of the brain itself and is most commonly caused by viral infection (especially of the herpes simplex virus type 1 in the UK). It is rarely caused by autoimmune disease such as NMDA receptor antibody encephalitis. The patient presents with confusion, headache, altered mental status, and seizures, in contrast to meningitis which more commonly presents with headache, fever, and neck stiffness. The best investigation for encephalitis is a lumbar puncture, which may show pleocytosis in viral encephalitis and antibodies in autoimmune disease. If the diagnosis is clinically obvious, treatment should supersede the lumbar puncture and use intravenous acyclovir and immunotherapy if autoimmune disease is the cause.

10) Correct answer: B

This child is presenting with benign rolandic epilepsy, also called epilepsy with centrotemporal spikes, which is a type of benign seizure that usually resolves in adolescence and hence does not usually require treatment. It consists of tonic-clonic seizures during sleep, with abnormal sensations on the face and the tongue. An EEG may show spike and wave morphology over the centrotemporal (or rolandic) area of the brain. Treatment is usually conservative as it is often benign and subsides as the child grows older.

For the different kinds of childhood epilepsy syndromes and seizure types, please see Paper 1, Question 20, Page 7.

11) Correct answer: D

Acute delirium is the most likely diagnosis. Also known as the acute confusional state, it is defined as acute alteration of consciousness and cognition level with reduced ability to focus, sustain, or shift attention. Risk factors include increased age (>1/3rd of general admission patients over the age of 70 have it), recent surgery, drugs, infection (most commonly a urinary tract infection), or displacement from usual settings (e.g., being in hospital, changing beds and wards). It develops over a short period and fluctuates during the day. It is a serious diagnosis that is often missed, with a risk of dying twice higher than average in the sixth month after an episode.

Management involves treating the source of delirium (e.g., infection) and conservative measures such as keeping the patient's room well-lit and furnished with clocks, reminding them of the date, and being reassuring and supportive. In cases of acute agitation, haloperidol or another short-term antipsychotic can be considered in the absence of any contraindications.

There is no clinical or medical history of Parkinson's, so drug withdrawal is less likely and new onset dementia would present more slowly and not over a few hours. There is also no history of alcohol misuse or malnutrition, so Wernicke's encephalopathy is less likely, and the patient lacks the classical features of Lewy body dementia (Parkinsonism, visual hallucinations, sleep disturbances, fluctuating cognition).

12) Correct answer: E

This lady has syringomyelia, the development of a cystic cerebrospinal fluid-filled cavity (syrinx) in the spinal cord. This most commonly occurs at the C5–C8 level and includes the classic symptoms of altered pain and temperature in a 'cape' distribution, as well as wasting of the small muscles of the hands. It is often bilateral. The only association is a Chiari malformation (Paper 3, Question 27, Page 41), whereby parts of the cerebellum protrude down into the foramen magnum, causing symptoms. MRI of the spine is the investigation of choice, which should demonstrate if the syrinx and Chiari malformation is present, and management Is based on the cause, such as surgical treatment of a Chiari malformation.

13) Correct answer: E

The correct answer to this question is anterograde amnesia, which refers to the inability to retain NEW information. Retrograde amnesia is the inability to recall events BEFORE the event or condition started, and both occur in Korsakoff's psychosis. This is a result of chronic thiamine deficiency, which is most commonly caused by low dietary intake (e.g., from chronic alcoholism, severe malnutrition), severe vomiting, and gastric band surgery.

There is destruction of the mamillary bodies in the brain, which causes memory disturbances. Another unique feature of Korsakoff's psychosis is confabulation — false perception and memories on direct questioning — making the patient seem as though they are 'making things up'. Treatment is with urgent thiamine replacement, but Korsakoff's psychosis when present indicates long-term damage and is often irreversible.

Wernicke's encephalopathy is acute thiamine deficiency and manifests with the triad of ataxia, ophthalmoplegia, and neurocognitive dysfunction (confusion, stupor). The key idea with Wernicke's is that thiamine replacement is very urgent, as it is in theory a reversible encephalopathy.

14) Correct answer: C

This patient has meralgia paraesthesia, a neuropathic pain caused by compression of the lateral cutaneous nerve of the thigh. It is linked to 2 things, obesity and diabetes, and this patient has both. It is described as a 'stinging' or 'burning' pain that runs across the anterolateral surface of the thigh in line with the nerve's distribution. Treatment is with adequate control of diabetes and, if severe, neuropathic pain medication (e.g., amitriptyline, duloxetine).

The other most sensible diagnosis here is diabetic amyotrophy, a severely painful condition with wasting of the quadriceps muscle, linked to poor control of diabetes. However, the 'stinging' pain with paraesthesia and obesity sways the diagnosis more to meralgia paraesthesia. Peripheral neuropathy secondary to diabetic amyotrophy would manifest in the limb extremities such as the feet, and may present with associated sequelae such as a foot ulcer, altered sensation, or a severely deformed foot due to damage accumulated from absent sensation (Charcot or concave foot). Trochanteric bursitis is more common in runners and can cause a similar pain, but given the obesity, poorly controlled diabetic amyotrophy, and neuropathic pain description, it is most likely meralgia paraesthesia.

15) Correct answer: A

The most likely diagnosis is benign essential tremor because the tremor is not resting, he gets better with alcohol, and his young age presenting with a tremor makes it more likely than

Parkinson's (although benign essential tremor is most common in people aged 40 and older). Familial Parkinson's syndromes do exist, but this is rare and a more significant family history would be expected to consider this as a potential diagnosis (a grandparent getting diagnosed age 70 is not uncommon). A rubral tremor (also called a Holmes tremor) is due to a lesion in the cerebellar peduncle, is a resting and intention tremor with sometimes irregular amplitude, and is linked to multiple sclerosis.

As the diagnosis suggests, the condition is benign, not linked to any other neurological conditions, and can subside with time.

16) Correct answer: C

The first line management for distressing benign essential tremor is propranolol or primidone. Although alcohol may help with symptoms, for obvious reasons it is not recommended for first line treatment!

17) Correct answer: D

Stroke, tumours, and multiple sclerosis are all causes of upper motor neuron examination findings, so the answer is between bulbar and pseudobulbar palsy. Lower motor neuron signs are seen in bulbar palsy, and the differences are illustrated in the table below. If you have to remember anything, just know that bulbar palsy causes lower motor neuron signs, in particular the tongue (flaccid, wasting/fasciculations), while pseudobulbar palsy does the opposite (stiff and spastic, brisk reflexes). The most common causes of bulbar palsy are motor neurone disease, poliomyelitis, and Guillain-Barré syndrome. The most common causes of pseudobulbar palsy are stroke, multiple sclerosis, and motor neurone disease.

Motor neurone disease can cause both bulbar and pseudobulbar palsy, which makes sense because it affects both upper and lower motor neurons!

Feature	Bulbar palsy	Pseudobulbar palsy
Type of lesion/signs	Lower motor neuron	Upper motor neuron
Location of lesion	Medulla	Bilateral, mostly internal capsule
Causes	Motor neurone disease, poliomyelitis, Guillain-Barré syndrome, myaesthenia gravis	Bilateral Stroke, motor neurone disease, multiple sclerosis
Tongue	Flaccid, fasciculations	Small, stiff, and spastic
Jaw jerk	Normal or absent	Brisk
Effect	Normal effect	Emotionally labile

*Source: 250 Cases in Clinical Medicine, 5th Edition (2019), Crash Course General Medicine (2018), and Neurology (2019)

18) Correct answer: E

Tuberous sclerosis is an autosomal dominant inherited disorder and can be remembered by the clinical triad of intellectual disability, intractable epilepsy, and facial angiofibromas (adenoma sebaceum — a benign tumour made up of blood vessels and connective tissue).

Skin features include facial angiofibromas (adenoma sebaceum), depigmented spots on the torso (ash leaf macules), and rough 'shagreen' patches over the lower back.

Apart from intellectual disability and epilepsy, the other features include brain tumours (most commonly giant cell astrocytoma), cortical and subependymal hamartomas, and cysts or tumours affecting the kidneys, muscles, and lungs.

Neurofibromatosis type 1 can be remembered as having 'Lisch' nodules in the eyes (iris hamartomas), axillary freckling, café au lait spots, and neurofibromas, as well as optic gliomas (optic nerve tumour).

Neurofibromatosis type 2 would have the oh-so-classic bilateral vestibular schwannomas, and they may also present with cataracts and multiple meningiomas.

Ohtahara syndrome, a very rare cause of epilepsy and early death in children, is a progressive encephalopathy that shows 'burst suppression' activity on the EEG (I wouldn't study this any further).

Sturge-Weber syndrome will present with a port wine stain, fragile blood vessels, and ocular disorders such as glaucoma.

19) Correct answer: E

Glioblastoma is a grade 4, aggressive glioma (brain tumour of glial cells) that carries a poor prognosis. It is highly vascular, often has areas of necrosis that will be found on pathology reports, and may even be evident on imaging. There is often brain invasion, and the tumour can invade the corpus callosum and adjacent structures. Treatment is with the triad of maximal surgical resection, adjuvant radiotherapy (after surgery), and temozolomide (a chemotherapy drug used only for glioblastoma).

Meningioma might be calcified and would more likely be a benign lesion; haemangioblastoma occurs in young patients and is thus unlikely in an adult although it will be vascular; an anaplastic astrocytoma may display these features but is a grade 3 glioma (less aggressive than a glioblastoma); and a cavernoma is a collection of benign blood vessels that would be evident on imaging and is not technically a brain tumour.

20) Correct answer: A

Bitemporal hemianopia describes loss of the outer (temporal) visual fields for each eye, creating 'tunnel vision'. This is due to lesions of the optic chiasm, or the part where the optic nerves cross over with each other. Causes of bitemporal hemianopia include pituitary adenomas and craniopharyngiomas (mainly affecting children).

An optic nerve glioma would cause unilateral blindness or loss of vision, while a stroke would cause homonymous hemianopia (loss of the lateral half of vision on the side contralateral to the stroke and loss of the medial half of vision on the same side as the stroke).

An occipital cortex lesion would cause homonymous hemianopia with macular sparing, which is the same as homonymous hemianopia but with a region of central spared vision.

See Paper 1, Question 36, Page 12 for a full diagram of different patterns of visual loss.

21) Correct answer: C

This patient is in a persistent vegetative state, because they still have sleep-wake cycles which excludes coma or brainstem death, they do not make any voluntary eye movements like blinking which rules out locked in syndrome, and they do not show brief episodes of higher consciousness level which would be consistent with a minimally conscious state. Knowing these key distinguishing features is important, and they are summarised in the table below:

Feature	Purposeful response to stimuli	Behavioural arousal, sleep wake cycles	Brainstem reflexes	Eye opening	Facial and vocal expression
Coma	No	No	Yes	No	No
Persistent vegetative state	No	Yes	Yes	Yes	Sometimes (may smile or cry)
Minimally conscious state	Sometimes	Yes	Yes	Yes	May be purposeful
Locked in syndrome	No	Yes	Yes	Yes	Sometimes (may grunt or smile)
Brainstem death	No	No	No	No	No

22) Correct answer: B

This patient has a GCS of 6 and should therefore be intubated, because when a patient's level of consciousness drops to a GCS of 8 or less, they are generally unable to maintain their own airway. This can be remembered as 'GCS 8, intubate'. All of the other options are not as suitable because a needle or surgical cricothyrotomy is only a temporary solution, while a nasopharyngeal airway is not a definitive airway and may be contraindicated if the patient has a basal skull fracture, which is entirely possible given the obvious head injury after the road traffic accident. This should be performed by an experienced anaesthetist or emergency clinician. This will also help to reduce intracranial pressure and stabilise the patient in the event that surgery or critical care intervention is needed.
Source: Advanced Trauma Life Support, 9th Edition.

23) Correct answer: B

The most commonly affected vertebrae in malignant spinal cord compression (MSCC) is the thoracic vertebrae (70% overall), simply because there are more of them. The lumbosacral vertebrae makes up 20% while the cervical vertebrae accounts for 10% (the least common, but potentially the most serious). Management involves urgent MRI within 24 hours if MSCC is suspected, with a view to using radiotherapy or surgical decompression depending on patient age and clinical status. Dexamethasone 16 mg should be given immediately unless contraindicated.

For a detailed explanation of MSCC, See Paper 1, Question 32, Page 11.

24) Correct answer: D

This patient has unfortunately suffered an intracerebral haemorrhage as a result of an arteriovenous malformation. This is the most likely diagnosis because although she describes a thunderclap headache before her seizure, which could represent a subarachnoid haemorrhage, the CT scan reveals no blood in the subarachnoid space, making this less likely. The MR angiography scan, which analyses blood vessels, also reveals torturous vessels and not an aneurysm, suggesting some kind of malformation. A cavernoma is a tangled mass of abnormal blood vessels and vascular channels but is usually occult on angiography, is less likely to present with a haemorrhage, and is not diagnosed by the Spetzler-Martin classification, which is how arteriovenous malformations are classified (that's all you need to know, you don't need any more than that!).

Arteriovenous malformations are intracranial tangled masses of pial blood vessels (nidi), and blood is shunted from arteries to veins. Many patients are asymptomatic, but they can become symptomatic and are associated with high mortality and morbidity causing haemorrhage, epilepsy, and focal neurological deficit. The chances of an arteriovenous malformation haemorrhaging is approximately 2–4% per year. Diagnosis is by CT or MRI angiography which can identify the abnormal blood vessels. Treatment can be conservative if the patient is asymptomatic, otherwise it can be a combination of surgical removal, using radiosurgery (SRS), or embolization as a neuroradiology interventional procedure.

25) Correct answer: B

Urea and electrolytes is the correct answer here, specifically sodium levels. This is because one of the complications of subarachnoid haemorrhage is hyponatraemia, which is due to the syndrome of inappropriate antidiuretic hormone secretion in response to the event, which leads to excess water retention with resulting low sodium levels. Therefore, sodium levels should be monitored in the immediate period after a subarachnoid haemorrhage.

Other complications of subarachnoid haemorrhage include cerebral artery vasospasm (prevented or treated with a calcium channel blocker called nimodipine), hydrocephalus (enlargement of the ventricles of the brain due to bleeding into the ventricles), seizures, and death if severe.

26) Correct answer: C

This is an imaging question, so it is important to understand the different kinds of neuroimaging and when they should be used. All you need to know about neuroimaging is summarised in the table below:

Imaging feature	Info	Good for
CT head scan	Basic scan, good for acute pathologies, less detail than MRI	Acute pathologies: Head injury Acute stroke Subarachnoid haemorrhage MRI contraindicated (e.g., claustrophobic, metallic objects)
MRI brain scan	More detailed than CT, good for everything except calcification	Brain tumours Any detailed structure Gadolinium contrast improves detection of tumours
CT/MR angiography	Dye injected into the leg to look at blood vessels	Aneurysms
Cranial ultrasound scan	Scan only used in infants (as it allows seeing through open fontanelles and does not involve radiation)	Infants Hydrocephalus
Lumbar puncture	Needle into the subarachnoid space allows the cerebrospinal fluid to be analysed	Meningitis Subarachnoid haemorrhage (done 12 hrs after symptoms if CT scan is negative) Idiopathic intracranial hypertension
Electroencephalogram	Electrodes put on the scalp to analyse brain activity	Epilepsy
PET CT scan	Metabolic scan that detects glucose, good for tumours	Not very accessible, LOTS of radiation dose

27) Correct answer: A

This patient has a Chiari malformation as evidenced by the occipital headache that worsens when intracranial pressure is increased (e.g., by a headache or lying flat), the risk factor of spina bifida (patients with this are at increased risk of having a Chiari), and the imaging showing enlarged cerebellar tonsils compressing the foramen magnum, which is the classical radiological feature.

A Chiari malformation is a group of posterior fossa brain abnormalities causing herniation or displacement of the cerebellar tonsils through the foramen magnum (the connection between the brain and spinal cord), leading to compression and subsequent symptoms. The most common symptoms are suboccipital headaches and neck pain. Risk factors include myelomeningocele (spina bifida) and syringomyelia.

Patients often need surgical decompression to relieve pressure on the spine, and this can be achieved by a foramen magnum decompression operation.

The patient's imaging does not reveal a brain tumour, she is not obese which makes idiopathic intracranial hypertension less likely, she does not have a history of rheumatoid arthritis, and she has headache — not neck issues — which rules out atlantoaxial subluxation.

28) Correct answer: E

Dementia, gait ataxia, and urinary incontinence? Think normal pressure hydrocephalus. This man's dementia may be treatable, and he needs a referral to a neurologist for further investigations. See Paper 1, Question 12, Page 4 for a full explanation of normal pressure hydrocephalus.

29) Correct answer: B

A common side effect of dopamine agonist drugs is gambling disorder, impulsivity, and hypersexuality due to the increase in dopamine levels. Postural hypotension is a characteristic side effect of levodopa specifically, which is also used to treat Parkinson's. Diarrhoea is a side effect of donepezil, an acetylcholinesterase inhibitor used to treat Alzheimer's disease. Finally, reduced seizure threshold is a side effect of clozapine, an atypical antipsychotic used in refractory schizophrenia.

30) Correct answer: D

The correct answer is methylprednisolone. This patient is having an acute exacerbation of her multiple sclerosis, and the treatment of acute exacerbations is steroids with pulsed intravenous methylprednisolone being used most frequently to acutely reduce the immune response.

Acetazolamide is a carbonic anhydrase inhibitor used in acute glaucoma treatment. Natalizumab and alemtuzumab are monoclonal antibody treatments used for refractory multiple sclerosis. Glatiramer acetate is used to reduce the frequency of relapses in relapsing-remitting multiple sclerosis. Natalizumab has a unique side effect of causing progressive multifocal leukoencephalopathy, a demyelinating brain disorder linked to long-term immunosuppression. Some common side effects of neurological drugs are listed here:

Medication type	Examples	Used for	Side effects
Dopamine agonists	Ropinirole	Parkinson's	Hypersexuality, gambling disorders
Levodopa	Levodopa, sinemet (combination of levodopa and carbidopa)	Parkinson's	Postural hypotension
Acetylcholinesterase inhibitors	Dementia, myasthenia gravis	Donepezil, galantamine, rivastigmine, pyridostigmine	Diarrhoea (donepezil)
Osmotic diuretics	Mannitol	Acutely raised intracranial pressure	Diuresis
Calcium channel blockers	Nimodipine	Subarachnoid haemorrhage (prevents vasospasm)	n/a

31) Correct answer: A

This patient has had a focal seizure with preserved awareness. The history is classic of a focal seizure, which is localised to one part of the brain, so it includes twitching, weakness, and stiffness, most commonly of one part of the limb or body. In addition, the patient can recall the events and is therefore 'aware' throughout. The classification of seizures has recently changed, and now complex partial seizure is frequently referred to as a focal seizure with impaired awareness.

A table summarising the new seizure classification is shown below:

Seizure type (new classification)	Old classification equivalent	Features
Focal (aware)	Simple partial	Jerking/twitching/stiffening movements If non-motor: sensation, emotions
Focal (impaired awareness)	Complex partial	Impaired awareness, automatisms like lip smacking, strange behaviours
Generalised Motor (tonic-clonic)	Tonic-clonic	Tonic phase of stiffness, followed by whole body jerking with loss of consciousness
Generalised non-motor (absence)	Absence	Occurs in children, often with 'vacant' expression and staring into space for a few minutes, inability to remember episodes

32) Correct answer: C

This is a tricky diagnosis, but the most likely one is a medication overuse headache. The features are not typical of migraine (e.g., no auras or photophobia), and the patient found that starting medications at a young age helped and has likely continued to use them despite not having symptoms, leading to her developing a medication overuse headache. To diagnose this, a patient must have a headache occurring on 15 or more days/month, whilst being on headache medication for more than 15 days/month, for more than 3 months. Treatment involves slowly withdrawing all medications to see if doing so has a benefit.

33) Correct answer: B

Prolactin can be used if tested within 30 minutes to separate a seizure from a psychogenic (pseudo) seizure. It is historically raised in seizures and is less likely to be raised in psychogenic seizures, so this is the test you would order. Lactate is more useful in diagnosing sepsis, mast cell tryptase is often used to help in the diagnosis of an anaphylactic reaction, and ferritin is sometimes used as a marker of inflammation (as it is an acute phase protein). Electrolytes can be a cause of seizures and should therefore be requested in seizure patients, but not to differentiate an epileptic seizure from a psychogenic seizure.

34) Correct answer: B

Anterior cerebral artery strokes present with any of the following: Personality change, urinary incontinence, and weakness affecting the lower limbs more than the upper limbs.

Middle cerebral artery infarcts cause face and arm weakness that affects the arms more than the legs, as well as prominent speech disturbance due to the Broca's and Wernicke's areas being affected.

Posterior inferior cerebellar artery infarcts present with lateral medullary (Wallenberg's) syndrome, consisting of loss of pain and temperature on the same side of the face as the stroke and contralateral loss of pain and temperature on the body. The patient may also have Horner's syndrome, ataxia, and diplopia.

Posterior cerebral artery infarcts present with predominantly visual disturbances, often with 'macular sparing' (the central part of vision is often preserved) due to the macula having a dual blood supply.

Lacunar artery strokes present with one of: motor deficit, sensory deficit, and ataxic hemiparesis.

35) Correct answer: A

The vitamin he is deficient in is thiamine (vitamin B1). This vitamin is heavily involved in brain metabolism and acute or chronic deficiency as seen in excessive alcohol consumption due to reduced nutritional intake, and excess vomiting and starvation can lead to the destruction of mamillary bodies involved in memory processing. Acutely, this leads to Wernicke's encephalopathy, a clinical triad of confusion, ataxia, and altered conscious level. This is reversible. If this deficiency persists, it can cause Korsakoff's syndrome, which leads to permanent memory loss.

Vitamin B3 (niacin deficiency) causes pellagra, which can be remembered by the 'Casal necklace', an erythematous pigmented rash in the distribution of a collar, and the 3 D's: **D**ementia, **D**iarrhoea, and **D**ermatitis.

Vitamin B12 deficiency causes subacute combined degeneration of the cord, where you get destruction of the white matter tracts leading to sensory deficits, weakness, ataxia, and gait disturbance, as well as mixed upper motor neurone signs (e.g., extensor plantar response) and lower motor neurone signs (e.g., absent knee reflexes).

See Paper 4, Question 16, Page 52 for a more detailed explanation of subacute combined degeneration of the cord.

36) Correct answer: C

This patient has had a stroke, and thus needs lifelong medication to prevent further strokes (secondary prevention). The standard of care for stroke prevention after a stroke or transient ischaemic attack is now clopidogrel. However, this patient has an allergy to clopidogrel, in which case modified release dipyridamole and aspirin should be commenced. High-dose aspirin (300 mg) is typically used for the first two weeks after a stroke before switching to 75 mg, but it is 2 weeks after his stroke and so this should be avoided. Apixaban is a factor Xa antagonist and direct oral anticoagulant that is used in stroke prevention, but this patient does not have atrial fibrillation and thus there is no indication to start it.

37) Correct answer: B

Gerstmann's syndrome is a clinical tetrad of finger agnosia, acalculia, agraphia, and confusion between the left and right sides due to a lesion or damage in the fusiform gyrus in the brain. I wouldn't learn anything else about this as it is HIGHLY unlikely to come up in finals examinations; just one for those who are very interested in neuroanatomy!

Weber syndrome simply describes a third cranial nerve palsy with contralateral hemiplegia, most commonly caused by a stroke.

Wallenberg (lateral medullary syndrome) is ipsilateral loss of pain and temperature on the face with contralateral loss of pain and temperature in the upper and lower limbs, often due to a stroke affecting the posterior inferior cerebellar artery.

Parinaud syndrome is a triad of upgaze palsy, unreactive pupils, and nystagmus, and is due to midbrain compression from either a tumour affecting the pineal gland (the one that produces melatonin) or a midbrain stroke.

Claude syndrome is a third cranial nerve palsy accompanied by ataxia.

Out of all these, lateral medullary syndrome is really the only one worth learning for exams if you ask me!

38) Correct answer: C

This is textbook meningitis, which is a medical emergency. The trademark symptoms of meningitis are fever, headache, and neck stiffness. The most common cause overall is actually viral, but bacteria can also cause patients to be acutely unwell and is the one with the most complications. Other symptoms are photophobia and general malaise, and patients with late-stage meningitis may have meningococcal septicaemia, where you get a purpuric, non-blanching rash (does not change when a glass is pressed on it). Other examination findings include Kernig's sign (extension of a flexed knee at the hip causes neck stiffness) and Brudzinski's sign (neck flexion leads to involuntary hip flexion), both indicating meningeal irritation. Cerebrospinal fluid for bacterial meningitis reveals increased cerebrospinal fluid pressure, presence of neutrophils or polymorphonucleocytes, and reduced cerebrospinal fluid glucose, and the Gram stain may show a bacterial organism. For a guide to cerebrospinal fluid in meningitis, see Paper 4, Question 35, Page 58.

Treatment is with immediate empirical antibiotic therapy, usually a third-generation cephalosporin such as ceftriaxone or cefotaxime.

Encephalitis would present with fever, headache, altered conscious level, and seizures, and cerebrospinal fluid might show a viral cause as opposed to bacterial.

Carbon monoxide poisoning could present with similar features, but the stem is lacking a history of others in the house having symptoms, a faulty boiler, or an obvious cause of carbon monoxide poisoning or pollution, and they have not mentioned carboxyhaemoglobin, which would be raised in a standard case of carbon monoxide poisoning.

Guillain-Barré syndrome would present with distal sensory loss and patchy weakness that evolves and ascends up the body, with loss of tendon reflexes on examination after a respiratory or diarrhoeal infection.

39) Correct answer: C

This scan shows a chronic subdural haematoma with all of the hallmarks — concave-shaped HYPOdensity (darker than the surrounding brain tissue) that crosses suture lines. Depending on patient symptoms, neurosurgical review with a view to drain the haematoma should be considered.

40) Correct answer: E

This scan shows a subarachnoid haemorrhage. This is because there is blood within the subarachnoid space (there is white near the edge of the brain that should normally be black), which commonly produces a 'starfish' pattern on CT scanning.

Practice Paper 4 — Answers

1) Correct answer: E

The correct diagnosis here is a low-pressure headache. This is caused by reduced circulating cerebrospinal fluid and is most commonly iatrogenic as a result of a procedure that removes cerebrospinal fluid, such as a lumbar puncture, which this patient has had. This reduces cerebrospinal fluid levels, which causes a headache that is characteristically worse when the patient stands up and is relieved by lying down. This can be thought of as the opposite to a raised intracranial pressure headache, where the headache would be worse when lying down, coughing, or straining, and is due to a lesion that causes raised intracranial pressure such as a brain tumour. Low pressure headache usually improves with time, but if it is disabling, there is some evidence that caffeine treatment can help (yes you heard it right; caffeine increases cerebrospinal fluid production apparently!).

Cluster Headache and post-coital headache diagnoses are not likely in this patient.

2) Correct answer: E

This patient has locked in syndrome, which is due to a lesion, infarction, or other damage to the pons and the midbrain region. As such, respiratory centres that initiate the breathing process are preserved, the patient will be conscious and have sleep wake cycles, and some eye movements may be preserved. The key thing to remember is that they have normal sleep wake cycles and may have preserved eye movements that allow for communication, just that all other voluntary muscle movement is lost. Prognosis is variable — some recover slowly — and treatment is mainly supportive.

Brainstem death, coma, persistent vegetative state, and minimally conscious state are summarised in Paper 3, Question 21, Page 39.

3) Correct answer: B

Disc herniation (prolapse) is caused by part or all of the nucleus pulposus (inner part of an intervertebral disc) protruding through the annulus fibrosus (outer part of the disc), which can compress the spinal cord and produce symptoms. It is a common presentation in general practice and can cause back pain and discomfort. Unlike mechanical back pain, the pain is usually burning or stinging, and there may be associated numbness or tingling that travels down the leg on the affected side. It is most common in the age groups of 30 to 50, and it is diagnosed using an MRI of the spinal area, usually the lumbosacral spine as the most commonly affected region is the L4/L5 and L5/S1 vertebrae. The other investigations would not help diagnose it except for a CT scan, which is used only if an MRI is contraindicated (see investigations guide) or in acute trauma (as it is much quicker than MRI).

Management of disc prolapse depends on the patient and severity of symptoms, but options include neuropathic pain medications and neurosurgical laminectomy (removal of excess prolapsed disc). 85% of cases will resolve within 8–12 weeks without any surgical treatment.

4) Correct answer: C

The correct answer here is a CT head scan within 8 hours because the patient does not satisfy any criteria for needing one within 1 hour (focal neurological deficit, GCS <13 or <15 2 hours after the injury, no features of a basal skull fracture etc), other than that he is over the age of 65 and has had a fall from a dangerous height (off a stepladder). These indicate that he needs a scan within 8 hours, even if he feels well and has no neurological deficits. As with all head injury patients, he should have regular neuro-observations and assessment of GCS as a precautionary measure.

See Paper 2, Question 28, Page 26 for a full explanation of CT head scan guidelines for head injury.

5) Correct answer: D

This patient has a left abducens (sixth cranial) nerve palsy. This is because an abducens nerve palsy affects the lateral rectus muscle, which moves the eye outwards when looking laterally or to the side. So, when the patient is asked to look in the direction of the side affected, the affected eye would remain stationary and be unable to move to that side, whereas the unaffected eye would be able to move on that side. Causes of an abducens nerve palsy are variable and include malignancy, trauma, and aneurysms.

A right-sided cranial nerve palsy would present in the same way, but the right eye would be affected and thus be unable to move to the right.

An oculomotor (third cranial) nerve palsy would present with a dilated pupil that is unreactive to light, ptosis due to palsy of the levator palpebrae superioris (muscle that lifts the eyelid up), and a 'down and out' pupil facing down and laterally.

A trochlear (fourth cranial) nerve palsy would present with the opposite of a third cranial nerve palsy, the patient may complain of 'vertical' double vision (2 objects seen on top of the other), and the pupil would be unable to move down and out when asked to, so it would remain in place while the unaffected eye would be able to move down and out as it supplies the superior oblique muscle that moves the eye in such a manner.

A diagram summarising this is shown below (note that the right eye is affected by all pathologies).

Cranial nerve palsy	Eye pattern	Diagram
Normal	n/a	
Oculomotor	'Down and out'	
Trochlear	'Vertical diplopia'	
Abducens	Lateral gaze restriction	

6) Correct answer: E

This patient has unilateral sensorineural hearing loss as suggested by the pattern of examination of Rinne's and Weber's tests. When you come across unilateral sensorineural hearing loss, think vestibular schwannoma or acoustic neuroma until otherwise indicated. This is a tumour of the Schwann cells lining the vestibulocochlear nerve, which is responsible for hearing and balance, and thus presents with unilateral hearing loss. An urgent MRI of the cerebellopontine angle (where the vestibulocochlear nerve arises from) and referral to neurosurgery is advised as these tumours can be removed, though hearing is often compromised as a result.

Hallpike's and Epley's manoeuvre would be used for diagnosing and treating benign paroxysmal positional vertigo; a CT head scan would be less effective than an MRI at delineating the tumour; and repeated hearing tests at 2 months would likely show the same pattern.

7) Correct answer: C

Yes, more dermatome questions. They are so commonly asked that it is worth going over them again and again! The medial side of the leg is supplied by L4, the big toe is L5, and the dorsum of the foot and the sole of the foot is S1. See the table below for a list of lower limb dermatomes you need to know:

Dermatome	Supplies
L1	Pockets
L2	Between pockets and knee
L3	Knee
L4	Medial side of calf
L5	Big toe
S1	Dorsum of foot and sole

8) Correct answer: E

This gentleman's ABCD^2 score is 5 because being over the age of 60 scores him 1 point, he is on antihypertensive medication so you can assume he has hypertension which would score him 1 more point, he had unilateral weakness so gets 2 points, his symptoms lasted 15 minutes (10-59 min) minutes which gets him 1 point, and he does not have diabetes. A score of 4 or higher indicates high risk of stroke, so he should be seen by a stroke clinician or team as soon as possible (within a few days) for evaluation and treatment initiation (usually of an antiplatelet medication for stroke prevention). The ABCD^2 score is used to evaluate the risk of a future stroke within one month of a transient ischaemic attack and is shown below:

Feature	Score
Age: >60 yrs	1
Blood pressure	
>140/90 or currently undergoing treatment for hypertension	1
Clinical features	
Unilateral weakness	2
Speech disturbance	1
Any other symptoms	0
Duration of symptoms	
0–10 min	0
10–59 min	1
>59 min	2
Diabetes	
Yes	1
No	0

9) Correct answer: A

This patient has a cerebral abscess as suggested by the classic triad of fever, headache, and neurological deficit. It is also supported by the fact that the patient is an Intravenous drug user as suggested by the track marks, which increases the risk, and the CT finding of a well-circumscribed mass with a ring border, which is classical of a cerebral abscess. Glioblastoma can also cause such CT findings, but in the context of an acutely unwell patient with fever and intravenous drug use, cerebral abscess is more likely.

Cerebral abscess is a collection of pus and fluid in the brain. It presents with the abovementioned classic triad of symptoms and can be caused by local spread of infection, such as from a paranasal sinus infection (the most common reported cause), otitis media and mastoiditis, or haematogenous spread from bacterial endocarditis. The most common causes are Staphylococcus and Streptococcus organisms.

MRI is the imaging method of choice for diagnosing cerebral abscess, which may reveal a ring-enhancing lesion in the brain parenchyma. Management is with high strength, long-term antibiotic therapy, which is often required to be given intravenously.

Progressive multifocal leukoencephalopathy is a progressive and fatal disease caused by the John Cunningham virus, which manifests symptoms in severely immunocompromised patients. It causes demyelination of the CNS and causes a wide array of presentations from cognitive impairment, ataxia, hemiparesis, and aphasia. It can be diagnosed by cerebrospinal fluid PCR, there is no effective treatment, and infection is often fatal.

10) Correct answer: C

The treatment of an acute cluster headache is with high flow oxygen and a triptan (e.g., sumatriptan). Prevention of cluster headache is with verapamil. For a full breakdown, see Paper 1, Question 16, Page 6.

11) Correct answer: B

This gentleman has unfortunately suffered a carotid dissection. This is likely given the fact that he now has neck pain and left-sided weakness, seemingly following a mild twisting of his neck from looking after his children, which is a common presentation. The only other plausible diagnosis from the list is tertiary syphilis, but this is not likely since there is no history of HIV or primary syphilis infection or any risk factors (e.g., risky sexual behaviour).

Carotid dissection is caused by a tear in the intima in the wall of the blood vessel, which can compromise blood flow to certain areas of the brain due to thrombus formation and cause a stroke. Risk factors are neck trauma such as a road traffic accident (which in some cases is seemingly trivial; e.g., a chiropractic manipulation!) and connective tissue disorders, such as Marfan syndrome and Ehlers-Danlos syndrome.

It is unfortunately a common cause of stroke in patients younger than 40.

Investigations are a carotid ultrasound and CT angiogram of vessels which is more accurate, and management is often with antiplatelets to minimise the risk of stroke or prevent another if one has already occurred.

Homocystinuria is an autosomal recessive inherited condition with thromboembolic tendencies, while CADASIL stands for cerebral autosomal dominant arteriopathy with subcortical infarcts and leukoencephalopathy. That's all you need to know; it most likely won't come up in finals.

12) Correct answer: C

The correct answer is listeria monocytogenes. This is suggested by the Gram stain, which reveals a Gram-positive rod (Neisseria meningitidis is a Gram-negative bacillus and E. coli is a Gram-negative rod). This makes it less likely to be Neisseria meningitis or E. coli, and the raised cerebrospinal fluid pressure and presence of neutrophils rule out viral factors. Tuberculosis is less likely because the glucose is not very low, and it is neutrophils, not lymphocytes, that were found. For interpretation of cerebrospinal fluid, see Paper 4, Question 35, Page 58.

13) Correct answer: D

The correct diagnosis is Bell's palsy. This is supported by lower motor neuron findings on examination (e.g., inability to close the eye on the affected side, loss of forehead wrinkles) as well as the sudden onset without other features of a stroke, such as speech disturbance and unilateral weakness.

Bell's palsy is a facial nerve palsy, thought to be caused by an inflammatory response to an agent (possibly viral infection) with paralysis of the facial nerve, which gives the characteristic signs. It is a lower motor neuron lesion and will specifically give signs like the inability to close the eye on the affected side, loss of forehead wrinkles, and hyperacusis (sounds heard much louder than they actually are).

Treatment is with high-dose corticosteroids as long as there is no contraindication, and most patients recover within 4–6 months, but for some patients the problem persists long term.

Ramsay-Hunt syndrome is a variant of Bell's palsy caused by the varicella zoster virus that affects the geniculate ganglion specifically, and therefore you get features of Bell's (the facial nerve palsy) and features affecting the ear, such as a characteristic painful, erythematous, blistering (vesicular) rash affecting the ear or the mouth. There may also be tinnitus or hyperacusis.

14) Correct answer: B

The correct answer here is a hemiplegic gait. This is where the limb is held in extension, and the affected limb swings around (i.e., circumducts) during the swing phase to prevent the feet from dragging. The most common cause is a stroke or other upper motor neuron lesion. An explanation of the different kinds of gait and what might be causing them are shown below:

Gait type	Gait pattern	Seen in
Trendelenburg (waddling)	Hip abductors are weak, so they do not stabilise the pelvis	Thyroid disease Cushing's syndrome Polymyositis and dermatomyositis

(Continued)

Gait type	Gait pattern	Seen in
Hemiplegic	Asymmetrical Affected limb held in extension Affected leg swings around (i.e., circumducts) during the swing phase to prevent feet from dragging	Stroke, space-occupying lesions
Parkinsonian (Festinant)	Festinant gait — short steps, shuffling Minimal arm swing Difficulty/hesitancy when asked to start, stop, or turn around May have associated tremor, rigidity, and bradykinesia.	Parkinson's disease, Parkinson's plus, drug-induced
Ataxic	Broad-based Unsteady Foot stamping	Cerebellar disease (stroke, space-occupying lesion) Bilateral: multiple sclerosis, alcohol, B12 deficiency, drugs (multiple sclerosis, alcoholism, phenytoin, barbiturates, lithium)
Neuropathic gait	Foot drop — weakness of dorsiflexion 'High stepping' gait to stop toes dragging along the floor Feet stamp on floor	Common peroneal nerve palsy L5 radiculopathy
Sensory gait (aka stomping gait)	Impaired proprioception, cannot see where the foot is Slams foot on ground to make sure it has hit	Tabes dorsalis Peripheral nerve disease: diabetes Vasculitis B12 deficiency Guillain-Barré syndrome Charcot-Marie-Tooth disease

15) Correct answer: E

This is classic hydrocephalus, evidenced by the hallmark features of enlarged head circumference, dilated scalp veins, and a 'sun-setting' appearance. Other features include enlarged or 'bulging' anterior fontanelles. The most likely cause in this case would be an intraventricular haemorrhage — a bleed that expands into the ventricles which blocks outflow of cerebrospinal fluid, causing dilatation of ventricles and hydrocephalus as a result. It is much more common in babies born pre-term due to fragility of blood vessels in the brain.

Myelomeningocele would present with a visible defect over the back containing parts of the spinal cord, while encephalocele would present with a large scalp protrusion, often filled with fluid and usually on the back of the head of the neonate. Although cerebral palsy is in some cases caused by an intraventricular haemorrhage, it is not the cause of the hydrocephalus.

16) Correct answer: D

This lady is presenting with subacute combined degeneration of the cord. This is the result of long-term vitamin B12 deficiency, most likely linked to her vegan diet, as meat products are a source of vitamin B12. This causes degeneration of some parts of the spinal cord, namely the dorsal column and medial lemniscus system and corticospinal tract. You get impaired proprioception and vibration, motor weakness, and a characteristic reflex pattern of weak or brisk knee jerks and the opposite for ankle jerks. Treatment is with replacement of vitamin B12, either through diet change or supplementation. It is usually reversible.

Inherited motor neurone disease is possible but highly unlikely; she is not taking any medication which rules out drug-induced peripheral neuropathy; tabes dorsalis is a manifestation of tertiary syphilis which occurs 20 years after a syphilis infection and is unlikely in a 21 year-old female; and she does not have diabetes which makes diabetic neuropathy a much less likely possibility, and it would present with 'glove and stocking' sensory loss most prominently in the hands and feet.

17) Correct answer: E

Hemiplegic migraine is the correct diagnosis because the person is having a migraine (dull headache) and has weakness, but detailed MR scanning is normal which effectively rules out a stroke. A stroke is also less likely given the age of the patient, and stroke is more likely to cause weakness than tingling. Either way, a patient with weakness and headache should be assumed to be having a stroke or transient ischaemic attack until proven otherwise, and in this case, this is effectively ruled out by the normal MRI head scan taken one day after presentation. An episode of multiple sclerosis is possible but does not explain the headache, while a subarachnoid haemorrhage could present as a stroke but the headache would be much more severe, and it would usually be picked up by the acute CT or MRI scan. Conversion disorder is possible but less likely given the headache.

Hemiplegic migraine is a rare phenomenon of migraine with associated one-sided weakness that can persist for days after the headache has settled. In 50% of cases, it is inherited in an autosomal dominant manner. Management is to first exclude a stroke, especially in a first presentation, followed by standard migraine treatment.

18) Correct answer: A

This consultant is asking about paroxysmal hemicrania, a rarer type of headache characterised by sharp stabbing pain, severe uniorbital pain, and autonomic symptoms such as conjunctival injection or lacrimation, miosis, and ptosis. It is known for its rapid responsiveness to a medication called indomethacin, and that's all you need to know for finals (see table below). Cluster headache would more likely involve a male patient with alarm clock headaches, lacrimation, and other autonomic symptoms; SUNCT is characterised by headaches that happen up to a hundred times a day in some patients, and is responsive to anti-seizure medications such as lamotrigine, topiramate, and gabapentin; a thunderclap headache is one that reaches maximum intensity within 5 minutes of starting; and the most serious diagnosis to exclude is a subarachnoid haemorrhage.

19) Correct answer: A

Dix-Hallpike to diagnose, Epley to treat. This patient has benign paroxysmal positional vertigo (BPPV) and is likely experiencing an acute attack. The Dix-Hallpike test is used for diagnosis, and this is done by placing the patient in a sitting position on a bed, positioning the head at 30°, and then taken to 30° below bed level. It is positive if vertigo is experienced after an interval period, and you should see nystagmus on examination. Nystagmus typically lasts 20–40 seconds and wanes with repeated testing.

Epley's manoeuvre is used to treat BPPV and is successful in 75% of cases. This involves lying patients down in a Dix-Hallpike position, turning their head 90° and it holding for 30 seconds, and sitting them upright whilst holding their head sideways.

A guide to BPPV, Meniere's disease, labyrinthitis, and vestibular neuritis is shown below:

	BPPV	Meniere's disease	Labyrinthitis	Vestibular neuritis
Key features	Sudden vertigo that lasts seconds, less severe on repeated movements, Dix-Hallpike to diagnose, Epley to treat	Tinnitus, vertigo, sensorineural hearing loss, ear fullness	Vertigo, nausea, and vomiting from viral infection, hearing loss	Vertigo, nausea, and vomiting from viral infection, NO hearing loss

(Continued)

(Continued)

	BPPV	**Meniere's disease**	**Labyrinthitis**	**Vestibular neuritis**
Hearing loss?	No	Yes	Yes	Yes
Time interval	Seconds	Hours	Days/weeks	Days/weeks
Cause	Crystals of calcium carbonate dislodged into semi-circular canals	Endolymph abnormality	?Viral infection	?Viral infection
Treatment	Epley manoeuvre	Low salt diet, vestibular sedatives (cinnarizine/ prochlorperazine), surgery	Acute attack: vestibular sedatives (prochlorperazine, cyclizine)	Acute attack: vestibular sedatives (prochlorperazine, cyclizine)

20) Correct answer: A

This patient has spastic diplegic cerebral palsy- this is because the weakness affects the two limbs specifically. The other subtypes of cerebral palsy are shown in the table below:

Cerebral palsy is defined as a non-progressive disorder of movement, posture, and tone due to a lesion or damage to the developing brain. Causes can be separated into antenatal, perinatal, and postnatal.

Treatments are mainly about managing function and improving quality of life, and includes physiotherapy, orthopaedic referrals, and baclofen to manage spasticity, while surgical options include selective dorsal rhizotomy — a procedure where the nerves are selectively removed to reduce spasticity and can improve quality of life if appropriate.

21) Correct answer: C

This patient has a relative afferent pupillary defect. This is when the eye dilates to light when it should not while performing a swinging light test (moving a torch from one eye to the other). Causes include optic neuritis, glaucoma, and optic nerve lesions such as tumours (most commonly meningiomas and astrocytoma).

Optic chiasm lesions would cause bitemporal hemianopia (tunnel vision); an occipital cortex lesion would cause homonymous hemianopia with macular sparing; and a lesion in the paramedian pontine reticular formation would cause one and a half syndrome, characterised by a combination of ipsilateral conjugate horizontal gaze palsy in one eye and ipsilateral internuclear ophthalmoplegia in the other.

22) Correct answer: B

This young man has post-concussion syndrome, most likely in part due to head injuries accumulated throughout his rugby career. Concussion is caused by trauma to the head and presents with memory loss after a minor or major head trauma. Post-concussion syndrome occurs after this, and symptoms include persistent memory deficit, irritability, migraine-type headaches, and inability to concentrate. Treatment is conservative management as 90% of cases have symptom resolution within 2 weeks, and symptoms may rarely persist for up to 1 year. All other answers are not really appropriate.

23) Correct answer: C

This lady has carpal tunnel syndrome caused by a narrowing of the carpal tunnel and pressure from the flexor retinaculum (a retaining band that runs above it) on the median nerve which passes through it, causing symptoms. These symptoms include numbness, paraesthesia, and weakness. The symptoms may be worse at night and are typically improved by waking up and shaking the affected hand ('wake and shake'). Risk factors include hypothyroidism, rheumatoid arthritis, acromegaly, and female sex. Examination often reveals wasting of the thenar eminence muscles of the thumb (as these are supplied by the nerve), and this is an indication for decompressive surgery. Two examination tests are associated: Tinel's test (tapping over the median nerve centrally just before the wrist) causes numbness and reproduction of symptoms, and Phalen's test (flexing the wrist for 30–60 seconds) causes numbness and reproduces the symptoms. (**T**inel's = **T**apping, **P**halen's = **F**lexing). Treatment is with managing symptoms (e.g., pain medication), wrist splint which extends the arm at night to prevent symptoms, and steroid injections (but symptoms recur in 80%). Final treatment is surgical decompression of the area, often by releasing the flexor retinaculum.

Ulnar nerve palsy would present with claw hand as innervation to the two lumbricals that extend the fingers is affected. If the lesion is at the elbow causing the ulnar nerve palsy, all ulnar muscles would lose innervation and thus clawing is absent. As clawing is therefore worse in distal lesions, it is called the ulnar paradox. You may also get wasting of the hypothenar eminence and dorsal interossei (small muscles of the hand).

Radial nerve palsy is also called 'Saturday night palsy', and it often occurs when a person compresses the radial nerve overnight (usually by leaning their affected arm over the back of a chair and sleeping on it). This causes loss of wrist extension and classically causes 'wrist drop'.

24) Correct answer: A

Tardive dyskinesia is defined as involuntary movements that affect the face, tongue, and mouth, and is linked to long-term typical antipsychotics used historically in the treatment of schizophrenia (e.g., chlorpromazine, haloperidol). The movements include lip smacking and dystonic grimacing. It is essential to avoid anticholinergics such as procyclidine, which is often used in other movement disorders such as dystonia but should be avoided in tardive dyskinesia because it will worsen the dyskinesia. A suitable alternative treatment is switching the medication to an atypical antipsychotic if this is not already done, but in many cases tardive dyskinesia is permanent.

Domperidone is an antiemetic, propranolol is a beta blocker, ezetimibe is a medication used to treat hypercholesterolaemia, and ciprofloxacin is an antibiotic; all of them carry no reason to be avoided in tardive dyskinesia.

25) Correct answer: E

The correct answer here is central pontine myelinolysis (contemporarily known as osmotic demyelination syndrome), a potentially life-threatening complication of correcting hyponatraemia (low sodium) too quickly. If too much fluids with sodium is given to correct this, it can cause shrinkage of brain endothelial cells, with immune response cells crossing the blood brain barrier, activating immune cells, and causing demyelination of the pons. Symptoms include motor abnormalities that progress to flaccid quadriplegia, respiratory paralysis, altered mental status, and coma. Risk factors include a change in serum sodium greater than 12mEq/L in 24 hours, alcohol abuse, hypokalaemia, and liver disease.

Progressive multifocal leukoencephalopathy is a rare complication of lymphoma, leukaemia, but most commonly immunosuppression (usually due to AIDS, organ transplantation, or patients taking disease-modifying drugs for multiple sclerosis). It is an infection of oligodendrocytes by the human polyomavirus 2 (John Cunningham virus) which causes demyelination of the white matter of the cerebral hemispheres. Clinical features are dementia, hemiparesis, and aphasia which progress rapidly in a patient with risk factors as above. The only treatment is reversing immunosuppression or treating the cause (e.g., AIDS).

26) Correct answer: B

The correct answer is Ramsay Hunt syndrome, a condition that is similar to Bell's palsy and is characterised by shingles in the geniculate ganglion, a facial nerve palsy identical to Bell's, and a characteristic vesicular rash around the external auditory meatus and/or soft palate, which differentiates it from regular Bell's. The reason for this is involvement of the geniculate ganglion, which supplies part of the ear. There may also be deafness and vertigo or unsteadiness. Treatment is usually with antiviral medication (acyclovir) and steroids, with complete recovery being less likely than Bell's alone.

27) Correct answer: D

This patient has cauda equina syndrome, which is a neurological emergency and can result in permanent neurological deficit (e.g., limb weakness, incontinence) if not treated urgently.

As the patient has presented acutely and has good functional status, urgent neurosurgical decompression is indicated in the absence of contraindications. See Paper 2, Question 24, Page 25 for a thorough explanation of cauda equina syndrome.

28) Correct answer: E

This is lateral medullary syndrome — loss of pain and temperature on the ipsilateral side of the face and loss of pain and temperature on the contralateral side of the body. The most common cause is a stroke, and it can also present with a sudden onset of vertigo, vomiting, and ataxia (posterior circulatory stroke symptoms). Medial medullary syndrome is remembered as having weakness unlike the lateral medullary syndrome, as well as paralysis and wasting of tongue muscles on the ipsilateral side with contralateral hemiplegia, and loss of vibration and joint position sense. It is caused by occlusion of the lower basilar or vertebral artery.

29) Correct answer: B

The correct diagnosis is central cord syndrome, because the lady has presented with a hyperextension injury (changing a lightbulb by elderly patients is a common exam scenario) and has examination findings of weakness in the arms but relative sparing of the lower limbs. See Paper 1, Question 40, Page 15 for an explanation of central cord syndrome.

30) Correct answer: C

Edrophonium (tensilon) test is the correct answer, because the patient has myaesthenia gravis and the way to diagnose this is by the tensilon test. This is where you give the patient a short-acting acetylcholinesterase inhibitor, which can increase acetylcholine levels temporarily. In a patient with myaesthenia gravis, there is often a transient improvement in weakness or ptosis. A patient without myaesthenia gravis would not have much difference. A CT scan of the thorax could be used to look for a thymoma (thymus tumours are seen in 10% of those with myaesthenia gravis), but would not reveal the exact diagnosis. The rest of the tests (e.g., MRI head scan, lumbar puncture) would not be useful for this patient.

31) Correct answer: E

This is Miller-Fischer syndrome, a variant of Guillain-Barré syndrome (GBS) characterised by ataxia, areflexia, and ophthalmoplegia. The weakness is also slightly different from GBS as it is often described as 'descending', which is the opposite of that of GBS, which is frequently described as ascending areflexic paralysis. Management is similar with conservative management, but if conditions are severe, intravenous immunoglobulin and plasma exchange can be carried out. Miller-Fischer syndrome has a higher mortality than GBS, but for exams should only be remembered by the triad of ataxia, areflexia, and ophthalmoplegia, with descending weakness. Patients with the Miller-Fisher variant also have anti-GQ1b ganglioside antibodies.

32) Correct answer: D

This question asks about the treatments for refractory Parkinson's outside of the traditional medications (e.g., levodopa, dopamine agonists). The correct answer is apomorphine. This is not actually related to morphine; instead it is a rapidly acting dopamine agonist used in treatment-resistant Parkinson's for 'on-off' periods, during which the patient does not have the effect of the Parkinson's medications and is frozen or slow ('off') versus having the medication and being hyperkinetic ('on').

The other treatments for Parkinson's that is resistant to medication include COMT inhibitors (stops the breakdown of dopamine by inhibiting the enzymes that break it down), MAO inhibitors (similar action, but limited by side effects), and surgery. Two surgical options include intrajejunal duodopa, which is an intrajejunal pump that releases dopamine, and deep brain stimulation, where an implantable device is inserted near the basal ganglia to reduce tremors. For finals, no further knowledge of these treatments is required; just know that they are available and can be used if medications have failed.

33) Correct answer: E

The impaired awareness, automatisms like lip smacking, and odd behaviours all suggest complex partial seizures. The metallic taste and epigastric sensation, often described as 'rising', indicate that this seizure arises in the temporal lobe and is either partial or focal. For a guide to other seizures, see Paper 3, Question 31, Page 42.

34) Correct answer: B

The correct amount of time to wait after thrombolysis before starting antiplatelet therapy in a patient with ischaemic stroke is 24 hours. After thrombolysis, a CT head scan within 24 hours is recommended, and if this is normal, patients are given aspirin 300 mg per day for 14 days, and then clopidogrel 75 mg indefinitely. If clopidogrel is contraindicated, aspirin 75 mg or modified release dipyridamole 200 mg can be used instead. For a detailed explanation of stroke, see Paper 2, Question 11, Page 20.

35) Correct answer: A

Based on the cerebrospinal fluid sample, this patient has bacterial meningitis. The features indicative of bacterial meningitis are high opening pressure, the presence of neutrophils (or polymorphonucleocytes), low glucose level, and a positive Gram stain, in this case a Gram-negative coccus with the most likely cause being Neisseria meningitidis. In viral meningitis, the opening pressure is normal or slightly raised, protein is often normal, white cell count is often normal and positive for lymphocytes only, and glucose is often normal. Tuberculosis meningitis is classified by very high opening pressure and very low glucose level, cryptococcal meningitis will produce a positive 'India ink' stain, and listeria meningitis will produce a Gram-positive rod on analysis and should be suspected in elderly patients presenting with meningitis.

A table summarising the different kinds of cerebrospinal fluid is shown below:

Feature	Normal	Bacterial	Viral	Fungal/ tuberculosis	Subarachnoid haemorrhage
Opening pressure (cmH$_2$O)	10–20	>30 (high)	Normal or mildly increased	High	High
Appearance	Clear	Turbid, cloudy	Clear	Fibrin web	Blood stained, yellow (xanthochromia) 12 hours later
Protein (g/L)	0.18–0.45	>1 (high)	<1	0.1–0.5	High
Glucose (mmol/L)	2.8–4.2	<2.2 (low)	Normal	1.6–2.5 (sometimes very low)	Normal
Gram stain	No organisms	Positive	Normal	Normal, may be positive on India Ink if cryptococcal or acid-fast bacilli if tuberculosis	Normal
Glucose-cerebrospinal fluid: serum ratio	>0.6	<0.4 (low)	>0.6	<0.4	Normal
White cell count	<3	>500 (raised) 90% PMN	<1000 (lymphocytes)	100–500	High

*PMN= Polymorphonuclear leukocytes

36) Correct answer: B

This patient has toxoplasmosis. This is caused by the parasitic infection toxoplasma gondii and is characterised by fever, confusion, and CNS signs. It is the most common cause of brain lesions in patients with HIV, which is heavily implied in this patient given the past history of tuberculosis, oesophageal candidiasis, and cytomegalovirus infections. Imaging classically shows intracerebral calcifications, which are pathognomonic of the diagnosis and hence distinguishing of toxoplasmosis.

CNS lymphoma would present with nonspecific symptoms. A patient with a history of lymphoma would have solid, periventricular space-occupying lesions.

A cerebral abscess is a possibility given the history, but the lesion would be cystic, round, and usually without calcifications.

37) Correct answer: C

This patient has myelomeningocele, the most severe type of spina bifida. This is because myelomeningocele is an open defect in the spinal canal, with the contents exposed without a covering sac. It commonly presents antenatally and is diagnosed on fetal anomaly scans or at birth with the deformity and neurological complications evident. The neurological complications of myelomeningocele include bladder and bowel dysfunction, as well as movement disorders like weakness. All spina bifida types are linked to folic acid deficiency, which is the only real risk factor. Treatment is with surgical correction often in the first few hours of delivery, and treatment outcomes are poor, with many suffering long-term neurological disability as a result of the defect.

Spina bifida occulta is a less severe form of spina bifida and presents asymptomatically on examination in an otherwise well child. A textbook exam sign is a well child with a 'tuft of hair' over the lumbar spine area. Later in childhood, children may get problems such as leg pain and recurrent urinary tract infections due to tethering of the cord (diastematomyelia).

Meningocele presents with a defect but less prominent neurological problems than myelomeningocele, and unlike myelomeningocele, the defect is often closed instead of open. Outcomes are good after surgical correction.

Encephalocele just describes extrusion of the brain and meninges through a midline skull defect, which can be corrected surgically. Patients often have underlying associated cerebral malformations.

Anencephaly refers to failure of development of most of the cranium and brain. Affected infants are stillborn or die shortly after birth. It is often detected antenatally, and termination of pregnancy is usually offered.

38) Correct answer: B

Brainstem lesions or pathology usually cause weakness of the ipsilateral side of the face and weakness of the opposite side of the body.

Lesions of the cerebrum would usually only affect one side, lesions of the spinal cord almost always affect both sides, ventricle lesions would just present with symptoms of raised intracranial pressure due to hydrocephalus (e.g., headache, nausea, vomiting), and cavernous sinus lesions would most likely present with cavernous sinus syndrome if symptomatic (see Paper 2, Question 26, Page 25).

39) Correct answer: B

This patient has hydrocephalus (dilatation of the ventricles that carry cerebrospinal fluid), which is suggested by the image showing massive lateral, third, and fourth ventricles. That is probably all you need to think of for hydrocephalus for exams: massive ventricles that will be visible to the naked eye. It is most commonly caused by obstruction of the ventricular system which drains cerebrospinal fluid, often due to a brain tumour, cyst, or structural defect. Treatment of acute hydrocephalus is with a ventriculoperitoneal shunt that allows the ventricles to drain excess cerebrospinal fluid into the peritoneum in the abdomen. Malignant middle cerebral artery syndrome would show a large, wedge-shaped area of infarct affecting the middle cerebral artery territory (most of the scan); a frontal space-occupying lesion is not visible on this scan; there is no air in the brain to suggest pneumocephalus; and a colloid cyst is not present.

Remember to describe the scan fully in an OSCE station (e.g., patient details, type of scan), and not just the diagnosis!

40) Correct answer: D

The patient is most likely in a long-term neurological rehabilitation ward because she suffered a massive stroke 6 months ago. The CT scan shows a large infarct in the middle cerebral artery territory and, as a result, the patient is likely to be left with significant neurological deficit. It is unlikely to be oedema as there is no space-occupying lesion, and it is too large and uniform to be vascular dementia (which would show one or lots of small hypodensities). If something is darker on a CT scan than the surrounding brain matter, it is an infarct or less likely fluid. The skull is completely formed, so she most likely has not had a decompressive craniectomy (operation to reduce massive brain swelling in stroke patients).

Practice Paper 5 — Answers

1) Correct answer: C

This patient has Todd's paresis, which refers to weakness of a limb after a seizure episode. It is not very common, but most frequently occurs in focal seizures and leads to a hemiparesis or hemiplegia that persists after a seizure (but can also include confusion, amnesia, and almost any deficit depending on the particular anatomic epileptic focus). Patients usually recover slowly, but it is often falsely interpreted as a stroke. Along with hemiplegic migraine, it can resemble a stroke and is one of the stroke mimics, which can be remembered by the four **S**'s: **S**eizures, **S**epsis, **S**yncope, and **S**ugar.

2) Correct answer: A

This patient has Lambert-Eaton myaesthenic syndrome (LEMS).

LEMS can be considered the twisted cousin of myaesthenia gravis, considering the fact that there is damage to the presynaptic calcium channels leading to weakness that improves after repeated movement. There is significant association with malignancy, usually small cell lung cancer. Management options include treating the malignancy, if appropriate, and 3,4 dipyridylamine. This is specific to LEMS as it indirectly increases calcium release, which prolongs the neuromuscular response.

This patient has stage IV lung cancer, which is very unlikely to be treated successfully with surgery and chemotherapy; prednisolone is not the best medication to use here; a thorax MRI may help with identifying a thymoma, which is sometimes seen in those with myaesthenia gravis; and pyridostigmine is an acetylcholinesterase inhibitor that is used for myaesthenia gravis.

3) Correct answer: E

The most likely diagnosis here is a cardiac arrythmia. The factors that suggest this are the symptoms of dizziness, palpitations, and syncope, which are suggestive of existing cardiovascular disease. Epilepsy is less likely given the lack of aura beforehand and the fast recovery without incontinence (these are all more likely in seizures). There is no postural change to suggest a vasovagal episode, and carotid sinus syncope is less likely here (a syncope that results from pressure on the carotid sinus, such as from wearing tight clothes like collared shirts).

4) Correct answer: B

Myaesthenia gravis is not a cause of Horner's syndrome, while the others — multiple sclerosis, lung cancer, carotid dissection, and cavernous sinus thrombosis — are. See Paper 1, Question 9, Page 3 for a detailed explanation of Horner's syndrome.

5) Correct answer: C

Donepezil classically causes diarrhoea (**D**onepezil = **D**iarrhoea). It is an acetylcholinesterase inhibitor that is used to reduce the rate of memory decline in dementia. It is most beneficial in mild to moderate dementia. For severe dementia, memantine can be trialled. Memantine is an NMDA (glutamate) receptor antagonist, as glutamate excess is thought to contribute to axonal damage in the process of Alzheimer's and exacerbate memory decline.

6) Correct answer: C

This patient has neuromyelitis optica, which is also known as Devic's disease. This is because the patient has symptoms of multiple sclerosis, but cerebrospinal fluid Is negative for oligoclonal bands — a hallmark of multiple sclerosis — and positive for anti-aquaporin 4 antibodies, which are diagnostic. The presence of bilateral optic neuritis also makes neuromyelitis optica a more likely diagnosis. Treatment with glucocorticoids, azathioprine or cyclophosphamide, and/or plasmapheresis seems to be equally effective for neuromyelitis optica than for multiple sclerosis.

Transverse myelitis describes an acute inflammatory disorder affecting the spinal cord with subsequent loss of function. Causes are usually part of a para-infectious immune response and may follow viral infection, such as HSV. It also occurs as part of multiple sclerosis and neuromyelitis optica. Treatment is with high-dose steroids or other immunosuppressive therapies.

7) Correct answer: A

This patient has dysarthria, whereby cognition (thinking processes) is normal but the muscles controlling speech are ineffective, causing slurred speech despite cognition being intact. Causes include stroke, space-occupying lesions, and any disruption to the speech pathway. A guide to the different kinds of 'dys-' terms used in neurology is summarised below:

Dysphasia: Disordered speech due to higher sensory dysfunction — can be categorised into Broca's (expressive) and Wernicke's (receptive).

Dysmetria: Lack of coordination of movement characterised by under- or overshooting. The classical example is asking the patient to touch your finger with their finger — and they will classically 'overshoot' or go past your finger.

Dysgeusia: Altered taste

Dysphonia: Altered voice (also known as hoarseness)

Dysphagia: Altered swallowing (gastrointestinal symptom!)

8) Correct answer: B

This patient has polymyositis, an inflammation of the proximal muscles (e.g., the shoulders, hips, glutes) due to infiltration of CD8+ T cells into the muscle, leading to necrosis of muscle fibres which causes weakness. Moreover, the patient does not have a skin rash or evidence of skin involvement, thus ruling out dermatomyositis. Patients may also present with fever, muscle pain, and tenderness.

The cause of myositis is unknown. Diagnosis is clinical, but creatine kinase may be raised and muscle biopsy and electromyography may show inflammatory changes. Management is with corticosteroids and immunosuppression.

Dermatomyositis has features of polymyositis with features of skin manifestations like photosensitivity, a 'heliotrope' rash around the eyes and a linear red rash over the knuckles and proximal phalanges (Gottron papules). In adults, it is often paraneoplastic (associated with malignancy).

9) Correct answer: B or C

This lady has evidence of peripheral neuropathy, based on the 'glove and stocking' sensory loss that is more prominent distally. The different causes of peripheral neuropathy should be remembered (which is the purpose for this strange question!) and include diabetes, subacute combined degeneration of the cord, alcohol abuse, and inherited disorders like Charcot-Marie-Tooth disease. Drugs can also cause peripheral neuropathy and is most commonly linked to anticancer drugs such as platinum compounds (e.g., cisplatin) and alkaloids (e.g., vincristine, vinblastine), so both B and C are correct! Other important drugs that can cause peripheral neuropathy are amiodarone (used for cardiac arrythmias) and nitrofurantoin (used for urinary tract infections).

10) Correct answer: E

This patient has internuclear ophthalmoplegia. This is a complicated disorder affecting the medial longitudinal fasciculus, a structure responsible for coordinating conjugate eye movements. In internuclear ophthalmoplegia, the affected eye (ipsilateral) has impaired adduction (moving the eye inward or towards the nose) with nystagmus when the contralateral eye is abducted. While very rare, it is more common in patients with multiple sclerosis (you may even see one as a medical student; I did!)- but really only one sentence is required to learn this. If a patient with multiple sclerosis has impaired adduction of one eye and nystagmus of the other — think internuclear ophthalmoplegia — and if you want the gold medal, know that it is caused by a lesion of the medial longitudinal fasciculus, a fibre tract responsible for eye coordination movements.

11) Correct answer: A

The correct answer here is procyclidine. This is because the patient has akathisia, which is motor restlessness that is often involuntary. It is usually caused by antipsychotic medications, and as this gentleman is currently undergoing active treatment for paranoid schizophrenia, he is most likely taking one. Akathisia describes a feeling of motor 'restlessness' and can be treated by withdrawing the medication or by using procyclidine, an antimuscarinic medication that can be used to reduce the symptom. The only other option is haloperidol, which might actually make the situation worse and thus should be avoided!

12) Correct answer: B

This patient has a strange constellation of symptoms and signs, especially given the recent stress of her exams, but normal examination makes a functional disorder a possible diagnosis. The consultant is testing Hoover's sign, which is elicited by asking a patient to extend the weak limb and then flexing the unaffected limb — it is positive if the patient automatically extends the 'weaker' limb. It does not confirm a functional disorder, particularly in this lady whose chief complaint is altered balance, but her history suggests it.

For an explanation of all the signs, see Paper 1, Question 26, Page 9.

13) Correct answer: D

The most likely diagnosis here is a vestibular schwannoma, based on the sensorineural hearing loss without other symptoms. It needs to be excluded urgently, and the best way to do this is an MRI head scan (specifically of the cerebellopontine angle). For a detailed explanation of vestibular schwannomas, see Paper 4, Question 6, Page 48. The other investigations listed, like the CT head scan, are less reliable and a general rule of thumb is that for acute problems like stroke, subarachnoid haemorrhage, or bleeds, a CT scan is the best investigation to choose, whereas for more subacute pathologies like tumours, an MRI is best.

14) Correct answer: B

This patient has pituitary apoplexy. This is because they have presented with thunderclap headache, which is a common presentation of a subarachnoid haemorrhage, but the history of having acromegaly and a previous pituitary tumour makes pituitary apoplexy more likely.

Pituitary apoplexy is an uncommon complication of pituitary tumours due to the occurrence of infarction followed by haemorrhage into the tumour. It produces sudden onset headache (often simulating the thunderclap headache seen in subarachnoid haemorrhage) with rapidly progressive visual failure and extraocular nerve palsies with acute pituitary insufficiency. It can often be managed conservatively with replacement of hormones and close monitoring of vision, but surgical decompression may be required if there is significant deterioration in vision.

Empty sella syndrome is often asymptomatic and describes a defect in the diaphragma sella with extension of the subarachnoid space. All or most of the sella turcica (where the pituitary gland lives) is devoid of apparent pituitary tissue, but pituitary function is usually normal.

Sheehan's syndrome is hypopituitarism due to ischaemia of the pituitary gland that occurs after a postpartum haemorrhage. It most commonly presents with failure to establish lactation at birth, amenorrhoea, or other features of hypopituitarism.

15) Correct answer: A

Yes, another question on subarachnoid haemorrhage and lumbar puncture timing — because this is very important and one of the most likely neurological questions to come up in exams, KNOW this pathway. The lumbar puncture would have an appearance of xanthochromia due to bilirubin detected in the cerebrospinal fluid, which gives a classical 'yellow' appearance. Bilirubin is formed as a breakdown product of red blood cells that enter the cerebrospinal fluid due to blood from the subarachnoid haemorrhage. This is why you have to wait 12 hrs after the onset of symptoms to perform a lumbar puncture — the red blood cells need time to break down first, otherwise the bilirubin that you test for may be falsely recognised as not being present. For more information on lumbar punctures, see Paper 4, Question 35, Page 58.

16) Correct answer: E

This patient unfortunately has brainstem death, and there are a few ways in which this can be diagnosed. Crucially, all brainstem reflexes should be absent. This includes: pupils fixed and unresponsive to bright light (and are often fixed and dilated), corneal reflexes absent, no vestibulo-ocular reflexes on caloric testing, no gag reflex, and spontaneous respiration absent. All of the other features identified are not tests used to indicate possible brainstem death.

17) Correct answer: B

This patient has Parinaud syndrome. This is a rare syndrome and is very unlikely to be required for finals, so feel free to skip here. It is caused by compression of the dorsal midbrain, which most commonly includes pineal region tumours and cysts. Other causes include hydrocephalus and tectal plate lesions. Parinaud syndrome has the classic triad of clinical signs: small irregular (pseudo-Argyll Robertson) pupils, supranuclear gaze palsy (inability to look up) and convergence-retraction nystagmus. Management is by treating the cause of the dorsal midbrain lesion; anything else is really not worth knowing!

Tertiary syphilis would just cause pseudo-Argyll Robertson pupils; a Holmes-Adie pupil describes an asymmetrical, often dilated pupil that reacts sluggishly to light in an otherwise healthy female and is thought to have a viral aetiology; and a Marcus Gunn pupil is one that dilates rather than constricts in response to the swinging light test, indicating an optic nerve lesion.

18) Correct answer: C

This patient unfortunately has Creutzfeldt-Jakob disease. This disease is very rare (occurring in approximately 1 in 1 million people) and is caused by a prion protein — a rogue protein that envelops and 'infects' other proteins in the brain, causing them to misfold. The exact cause is often unknown as most cases are sporadic, but it is sometimes passed to patients from contaminated meat (referred to as 'mad cow disease') or contaminated neurosurgical instruments. Creutzfeldt-Jakob disease is characterised by rapid memory dysfunction, personality change, general decline and death, usually within 18 months of diagnosis. On examination, startle myoclonus (electric shock-type movements) may be found. Unfortunately, there is no treatment for this disease, and most patients decline quickly and die within 2 years.

19) Correct answer: D

Benzodiazepines are GABA agonists and act on the GABA receptor to reduce depolarisation and hence an action potential. They can be used as antiepileptic drugs, antispasmodics, hypnotics, and sedatives. An example of a glutamate antagonist would be Riluzole, which is used in motor neurone disease.

20) Correct answer: A

This patient has presented with inferior quadrantanopia — this means that the affected area has to be the parietal lobe — because the upper optic radiation fibres that pass through the parietal lobe actually supply the lower visual field, while the lower optic radiation fibres that pass through the temporal lobe supply the upper visual field. If the lesion was in the temporal lobe, it would cause superior quadrantanopia (strange, I know). The fact that the visual loss is on the right side means that the opposite lobe of the brain must be affected, hence the answer being the left parietal lobe.

For explanations of visual fields and defects, see Paper 1, Question 36, Page 12.

21) Correct answer: E

This child unfortunately has Moya Moya disease. It is highly unlikely to come up in finals, so I would advise just knowing that it is a differential in any child with multiple ischaemic strokes. It is characterised by idiopathic narrowing of the intracerebral arteries, leads to strokes in children, and is more common in Japanese or Asian patients. That's all you need to know, but for the enthusiasts, there is a pretty cool neurosurgical operation you can do to help manage the condition (google 'EDAS Moyamoya').

CADASIL stands for cerebral autosomal dominant arteriopathy with small subcortical infarcts and leukoencephalopathy, and it is an autosomal dominant inherited condition causing transient ischaemic strokes, strokes, and dementia in young adult patients (usually around the age of 40).

Hurler syndrome is a rare, autosomal recessive lysosomal storage disease that usually presents within a few weeks of birth and causes cognitive impairment, heart disease, characteristic facies, and reduced life expectancy.

22) Correct answer: C

This patient has diabetic neuropathy. The reasons for this are the metabolic risk factors like raised BMI, presence of sensory loss in a 'glove and stocking' pattern (with symptoms more prevalent the more distal the limbs are), and the deformed foot — called a 'Charcot joint' — which happens due to altered proprioception and sensation, causing injuries to the foot over time due to misplacement. The presence of diabetic ulcers also increases the likelihood of diabetes being the cause of the patient's symptoms.

Patients' blood sugar should be controlled within a medical range (HbA1c of 48-53 depending on whether they are taking any hypoglycaemic medications) and managed from there. Other peripheral complications include foot ulcers, osteomyelitis (infection of the bones), and amputation of digits.

Buerger's disease (now known as thromboangiitis obliterans) is a non-atherosclerotic vasculitis that is linked to an inflammatory response in the arteries and usually affects male patients who are heavy smokers. Symptoms are associated with vascular compromise like intermittent claudication, rest pain, or tissue loss and frequently resolves on smoking cessation.

23) Correct answer: D

This young boy unfortunately has subacute sclerosing panencephalitis, a rare complication of measles that occurs many years after the initial infection. The exact nature of the disease is unclear, but patients usually present years after the illness in childhood and adolescence with intellectual decline, apathy, and clumsiness followed by myoclonus, ocular manifestations, and dementia. Regrettably, there is no treatment and most patients succumb to the disease within a few years.

24) Correct answer: C

Ah, the 'localising the lesion' question. Here is the guide. The correct answer is the pons — it is in the brainstem because you get ipsilateral symptoms on the side of the face to the lesion with contralateral weakness. For the pons specifically, the nerves affected are 5–8 (cranial nerves 3–4 arise from the midbrain, 5–8 from the pons, and 9–12 from the medulla), and as this patient has an abducens nerve palsy (sixth cranial nerve), the answer must be the pons.

25) Correct answer: C

Her GCS is 9. I have repeated a GCS interpretation question because it is important whatever your speciality is as a doctor (and I am running out of ideas at this point!). For GCS interpretation, see Paper 1, Question 8, Page 3.

26) Correct answer: A

The correct answer here is tuberous sclerosis, which is explained in Paper 3, Question 18, Page 38.

27) Correct answer: E

How you manage acute migraine is as follows: according to the latest NICE guidelines, the management of acute migraine involves a combination of an oral triptan and an NSAID, or an oral triptan and paracetamol. For people aged 12–17 years old, consider using a nasal triptan over an oral triptan. If these are not effective, consider a non-oral preparation of metoclopramide and a non-oral NSAID or triptan. For migraine, see Paper 2, Question 7, page 19.

28) Correct answer: B

This patient has progressive multifocal leukoencephalopathy (PML). This is a very rare demyelinating disease that is caused by reactivation of the John Cunningham virus and only affects immunocompromised patients, most likely those with HIV/AIDS or are immunocompromised due to leukaemia, post-transplants, or immunosuppressive medications (in particular natalizumab, a monoclonal antibody treatment for multiple sclerosis). It usually causes progressive general decline with altered mental status, motor deficits, limb and gait ataxia, and double vision being common. The only way to diagnose PML is by brain biopsy. Prognosis is poor and if untreated, PML is fatal within 6 months. Highly active antiretroviral therapy and steroids may prolong survival.

29) Correct answer: C

Unfortunately, Samira has Sheehan's syndrome, an ischaemic necrosis of the anterior pituitary gland that often occurs during childbirth. As the pituitary gland doubles in size during pregnancy and becomes highly vascular, any haemorrhage during childbirth can reduce blood pressure and blood supply to the gland, causing necrosis. It most commonly presents after a difficult childbirth, with the most common symptom being lactation failure due to prolactin deficiency followed by secondary amenorrhoea. Oestrogen replacement may be required, and depending on severity, replacement of all pituitary hormones may be required as well.
Source: Master Medicine: General and Systematic Pathology (2009)

30) Correct answer: B

The following questions (30–38) are shorter questions that overlap to some degree with questions in the previous practice papers.

The correct management of status epilepticus is intravenous lorazepam 4mg, which can be repeated once after 10 minutes if required. Buccal midazolam or rectal diazepam can be used if there is no intravenous access or the patient is in a remote location.

31) Correct answer: D

For migraine prevention, the first line is propranolol. If asthma, it is topiramate, but also remember that **T**opiramate is **T**eratogenic. Sumatriptan with high flow oxygen is for acute cluster headache, while verapamil is for prevention of cluster headache.
Source: https://cks.nice.org.uk/topics/headache-cluster/management/management/

32) Correct answer: A

Parkinson's symptoms, but autonomic symptoms (postural hypotension, erectile dysfunction, gastroparesis)? Think Parkinson's plus syndrome, specifically multiple systems atrophy. When eye movements are affected, think progressive supranuclear palsy.

33) Correct answer: C

No contraction = 0, flicker of contraction = 1, movement if gravity eliminated = 2, movement against gravity but not resistance = 3, active movement against gravity and resistance = 4, normal power = 5.

34) Correct answer: D

Head injury with loss of consciousness in a young patient followed by quick recovery and then a drop in GCS level? Think extradural haematoma until proven otherwise. Elderly or alcohol misuse plus trivial head injury? Think acute subdural haematoma. Cerebrospinal fluid rhinorrhoea, panda eyes, bruising over the mastoid process, and haemotympanum (bleeding from the ear)? Think basal skull fracture.

35) Correct answer: D

History of malignancy with new onset subacute neurological symptoms or signs? Think cerebral metastases.

36) Correct answer: C

Contraindications to lumbar puncture: space-occupying lesion on scans, signs of raised intracranial pressure (e.g., hypertension, bradycardia), cardiovascular instability, and known coagulopathy such as clotting or bleeding disorders.

37) Correct answer: B

If there is suspected spinal cord compression, first administer dexamethasone and lie the patient flat, and if the patient is fit enough and stabilised, refer them for urgent surgical decompression or oncology input.

38) Correct answer: D

Nimodipine is a calcium channel blocker used in subarachnoid haemorrhage to prevent vasospasm.

39) Correct answer: D

This scan shows an acute on chronic subdural haematoma. This is because acute blood (white) is present in a banana or concave shape, but there is also the presence of chronic blood (black) as part of the same haematoma. That means that this is an acute-on-chronic subdural haematoma, most likely the result of the patient's repeated falls. Options include conservative management or surgical drainage if there is midline shift on scans or if the patient is symptomatic (weakness or reduced GCS). See Paper 1, Question 38, Page 13 for more information on the different kinds of haematomas.

40) Correct answer: C

There is a large space-occupying lesion on this scan, evidenced by it being round, regular, and just a lesion! Differentials for any mass on an MRI head scan include tumours (e.g., meningioma, glioblastoma), cerebral abscesses (the lesion may be rounder and have a regular outline), and metastases (most commonly from lung cancer). Strange causes like infections and vascular pathologies (e.g., arteriovenous malformations, aneurysms, and inflammatory diseases like multiple sclerosis plaques) are also possible, but should only be mentioned in clinical exams after the most common causes! Further interpretation (e.g., area, extent of oedema) is most likely not required for medical school examinations.

One Sentence Summaries Index (in Alphabetical Order)

ABCD² score: **A**ge, **B**lood pressure, **C**linical features, **D**uration, **D**iabetes — to predict stroke risk after transient ischaemic attack.

Acute stress reaction: Stress++ event, numbness, detachment, and strange symptoms, resolve with support.

Akathisia: Motor restlessness, desire to move limbs constantly.

Alzheimer's disease: Degenerative disease due to Tau protein accumulation, hippocampus affected, short-term memory loss, treat with acetylcholinesterase inhibitors.

Anterior cord syndrome: Flexion injury, loss of pain and temperature with weakness worse in legs than arms.

Argyll Robertson pupil: Bilateral small, irregular pupil, fixed to light but constricts on convergence — think neurosyphilis!

Arteriovenous malformation: Congenital tangle of blood vessels, presents with bleeding or seizures.

Bamford (Oxford) stroke criteria: Unilateral weakness or sensory deficit, homonymous hemianopia, and higher cerebral dysfunction; LACS is 1, PACS is 2, and TACS is all 3!

Basal skull fracture signs: Cerebrospinal fluid rhinorrhoea, haemotympanum, raccoon or panda eyes, blood behind the ears (Battle's sign).

(Benign) Essential tremor: Benign tremor, family history, improves with alcohol, treat with propranolol or primidone.

Benign (Rolandic) epilepsy with centrotemporal spikes: Focal seizures during sleep or in the early morning, abnormal sensation on the tongue or face, most resolve by age 16.

Brain metastases: Any patient with cancer and new headache or raised intracranial pressure symptoms, most commonly from the lung > breast > melanoma > colon.

Brainstem death: No sleep-wake cycles or active breathing, fixed pupils, absent oculovestibular, corneal, cough, or gag reflex (rule out reversible causes first!).

Broca's (expressive) aphasia: Understands but cannot speak, appears frustrated, left frontal lobe (commonly due to stroke).

Brown-Séquard syndrome: 'One leg weak and one leg numb', spinal cord hemisection.

Bulbar palsy: Lower motor neuron lesion of the 7th to 12th cranial nerves, flaccid tongue and fasciculations, absent gag reflex or jaw jerk, caused by Guillain-Barré and poliomyelitis.

Carotid artery dissection: Cause of stroke in young patients, (trivial) neck injury causes tear à clot embolises and leads to stroke.

Carpal tunnel syndrome: Weakness, paraesthesia, Tinel's and Phalen's sign to diagnose, treat with conservative management → splints → steroids → surgical decompression.

Cauda equina syndrome: Back pain or sciatic pain with bladder or bowel disturbance OR bilateral leg pain OR saddle or genital sensory disturbance — urgent MRI to rule it out, surgical decompression needed!

Cavernoma: Benign collection of blood vessels, present with seizures — remove if symptomatic

Cavernous sinus thrombosis: Painful ophthalmoplegia, chemosis, and proptosis, caused by sinus infection or cancer spread.

Central cord syndrome: Hyperextension injury, weakness of the upper limbs but sparing of the lower limbs, most recover.

Central pontine myelinolysis (osmotic demyelination syndrome): Acute confusion and drop in GCS from rapid correction of hyponatraemia (brain swelling).

Cerebral abscess triad: Fever, headaches, limb weakness (intravenous drug use and immunocompromise) — scan shows ring-enhancing lesion, treat with antibiotics.

Cerebral perfusion pressure: Mean arterial pressure, intracranial pressure.

Charcot-Marie-Tooth disease: Autosomal dominant inherited peripheral neuropathy, pes cavus and champagne bottle legs present.

Chiari malformation: Enlarged cerebellum protruding through foramen magnum, posterior headaches or neck pain on coughing, treat with surgical decompression.

Claude's syndrome: Third cranial nerve palsy and contralateral ataxia (midbrain stroke).

Cluster headache: Males, restlessness with autonomic symptoms, O_2 and triptan acute with verapamil to prevent.

Cluster headache treatment: O_2 and triptan if acute, verapamil to prevent.

Coma: Lack of consciousness, no response to stimuli, no sleep-wake cycles, brainstem activity present.

Corticobasal degeneration: + Parkinson's + motor symptoms

Creutzfeldt-Jakob disease: Prion disease, rapid dementia, myoclonus, and death.

Cushing's triad for raised intracranial pressure: Hypertension, bradycardia, irregular respiratory pattern.

Degenerative cervical myelopathy: Weakness with loss of dexterity in the hands, older patients, decompressive surgery to stop progression.

Delirium: Acute alteration of consciousness, agitated, sleep-wake cycle reversal, reversible unlike dementia.

Dermatomyositis: Myositis plus heliotrope (violet) rash on eyelids with Gottron (violet) papules, think malignancy!

Diffuse axonal injury: Massive brain injury (e.g., decreased blood flow from cardiac arrest), diffuse white matter changes on scan, poor prognosis.

Encephalitis: Meningitis plus seizures and altered consciousness, HSV is the most common cause, treat with intravenous acyclovir (antiviral).

Encephalocele: Neural tube defect, brain goes through skull defect in neonates → surgery.

Extradural haematoma: Young patient with head injury, lucid interval, lens-shaped on CT scan (life-threatening).

Frontal lobe syndrome: Lack of executive function (planning, processing, words/speech, inhibition) — also known as dysexecutive syndrome.

Gerstmann's syndrome: Clinical tetrad of finger agnosia, acalculia, agraphia, and confusion between the right and left sides.

Giant cell arteritis: Elderly, headache with jaw claudication, scalp tenderness, and polymagia rheumatica require urgent steroids to prevent blindness!

Guillain-Barré syndrome: Ascending areflexic paralysis, previous campylobacter or diarrhoeal infection.

Glioblastoma: Grade IV brain tumour, horrible prognosis despite surgery, radio and chemotherapy.

Hemiplegic migraine: Weakness that persists after migraine, need to exclude stroke first.

Herniation (subfalcine): Movement of brain contents across the falx (due to mass effect from tumour or bleeding), often asymptomatic.

Herniation (tentorial/uncal): Dilated pupil and contralateral hemiparesis, from tumour or bleed pressing on the midbrain.

Herniation (tonsillar): Large mass causes cerebellar tonsils to go through the foramen magnum → breathing centres compromised.

Holmes-Adie pupil: Dilated pupil that is sluggish to light but sometimes accommodates, young females, benign finding.

Horner's syndrome: Ptosis, miosis, enophthalmos, facial anhidrosis (apical lung tumour is a common cause).

Huntington's disease: Alzheimer's disease disorder, exhibits anticipation, chorea, psychiatric disturbance, incurable neurological decline.

Hydrocephalus signs in an infant: Enlarged head circumference, bulging fontanelle, dilated scalp veins, 'sun setting' (child looks down).

Idiopathic intracranial hypertension: Young obese females, raised intracranial pressure and visual changes, treat with weight loss > acetazolamide > ventriculoperitoneal shunt.

Infantile spasms (West syndrome): 3–12 months old, 'salaam' attacks, resembles colic.

Internuclear ophthalmoplegia: Affected eye cannot adduct with nystagmus of the other eye — more common in multiple sclerosis and due to a lesion of the medial longitudinal fasciculus!

Intracranial hypotension: Often iatrogenic (lumbar puncture to drain the cerebrospinal fluid), headache worse when standing up, hydration and caffeine to treat.

Juvenile myoclonic epilepsy: Triad of myoclonic, generalised tonic-clonic, and absence seizures — adolescents, worse in the morning, sleep, and alcohol.

Korsakoff's syndrome: Anterograde and retrograde amnesia, confabulation (lying, making up gaps in memory), alcohol misuse → thiamine deficiency and mamillary body (memory) damage — IRREVERSIBLE.

Lambert-Eaton myaesthenic syndrome: Weakness that improves after repeated motion (autoantibodies vs presynaptic calcium channels) — common in small cell lung cancer.

Lateral medullary (Wallenberg's) syndrome: Posterior inferior cerebellar artery infarct, loss of pain and temperature on ipsilateral face and contralateral body.

Lewy Body dementia: Parkinson's with visual hallucinations, sleep disturbance, and fluctuating cognition.

Locked in syndrome: Brainstem damage resulting in damage to voluntary muscles — have sleep-wake cycles, are conscious, communicate with eye movements.

(Lumbar) Disc prolapse: Unilateral 'shooting pain' back → leg, 'sciatica' — conservative → neuropathic pain meds → steroid injection → surgery

Lumbar puncture contraindications: Raised intracranial pressure (hypertension, bradycardia), cardiorespiratory instability, coagulopathy.

Malignant middle cerebral artery infarction: Massive middle cerebral artery stroke with brain swelling, needs decompressive craniectomy to stop swelling.

Meningioma: Benign tumour of the meninges, grows slowly, often calcified, surgery if symptomatic.

Meningitis: Headache, fever, neck stiffness, photophobia — 3rd generation cephalosporin to treat.

Meralgia paraesthesia: Lateral cutaneous nerve of the thigh, poorly controlled diabetics — burning pain down lateral thigh — improves with diabetes control.

Metastatic (malignant) spinal cord compression: Any cancer patient with new back pain or neurological disturbance, lie flat and administer dexamethasone 16mg, neurosurgical or oncology referral.

Migraine: Headache, photophobia, females, 4-72hrs — management with propranolol or topiramate.

Miller-Fischer syndrome: Ataxia, areflexia, and ophthalmoplegia with descending weakness.

MRC grades of muscle power: 0 = no movement, 1 = flicker, 2 = gravity gone, 3 = not resistance, 4 = resistance but not full, 5 = full power.

Moya Moya disease: Child with repeated strokes, more common in Japanese children.

Motor neurone disease: Weakness, dysphagia, upper and lower motor neuron signs, incurable (riluzole improves survival by 3 months).

Myasthenia gravis: Muscle weakness or diplopia worse after activity, thymoma in 10% of patients, acetylcholinesterase inhibitors to treat.

Myelomeningocele: Open defect where the spinal cord is linked to folate deficiency, operated at birth, often associated with movement and bowel or bladder function problems.

Multiple sclerosis: CNS symptoms (optic neuritis, sensory/motor) separated in time and space — young females, relapsing-remitting the most common type.

Narcolepsy: Hypocretin deficiency — daytime sleepiness, cataplexy, hypnagogic hallucinations (when going to sleep), sleep paralysis.

Neurofibromatosis type 1: Autosomal dominant, neurofibromas, Lisch nodules, angiofibromata with brain tumours.

Neurofibromatosis type 2: Autosomal dominant, bilateral vestibular schwannomas with meningiomas.

Neuromyelitis optica (NMO, Devic's disease): Bilateral optic neuritis with spinal/CNS symptoms- similar to MS but anti-aquaporin 4 antibodies positive.

Normal pressure hydrocephalus: Wet, wacky, wobbly — urinary incontinence, dementia, and gait ataxia.

Panayiotopoulos syndrome: Benign epilepsy type, 1–5 years old, vomiting or autonomic symptoms during sleep, occipital spikes on EEG, remits in adolescence.

Parinaud syndrome: Dorsal midbrain syndrome — upward gaze palsy, pseudo Argyll-robertson pupil, and convergence retraction nystagmus.

Parkinson's plus syndromes:

Paroxysmal hemicrania: Headache with autonomic symptoms, similar to cluster headache, increased response to indomethacin.

Multiple systems atrophy: + Parkinson's + autonomic symptoms

Progressive supranuclear palsy: Parkinson's + eye movement problems and early falls

Drug induced parkinson's: Bilateral tremor, responds to medication withdrawal

Persistent vegetative state: No purposeful response to stimuli, still have sleep-wake cycles and brainstem activity.

Pituitary apoplexy: Haemorrhage from pituitary tumour mimicking subarachnoid haemorrhage with visual disturbance.

Polymyositis: Post-viral muscle inflammation, widespread weakness of proximal muscles.

Post-concussion syndrome: Headache, reduced concentration and memory, can lead to adverse mental health after concussion, most resolves.

Posterior communicating artery (PCOM) aneurysm: Painful third cranial nerve palsy.

Progressive multifocal leukoencephalopathy: Severely immunocompromised, progressive neurological decline, John Cunningham virus reactivation.

Pseudobulbar palsy: Upper motor neuron, no tongue wasting like in bulbar palsy, 'Donald Duck' speech, increased jaw jerking.

Psychogenic seizures/non-epileptic attack disorder: Eyes closed, quick recovery, crying or tearful after, different pattern of attacks.

Radial nerve (Saturday night) palsy: 'Wrist drop', cannot extend wrist after hanging arm off the chair whilst sleeping!

Raised intracranial pressure headache: Progressive, worse in the mornings and when lying flat, nausea and vomiting, may show papilloedema on examination.

Relative afferent pupillary defect: Pupil that dilates rather than constricts to the swinging light test — optic nerve issue.

Ramsay Hunt syndrome: Facial nerve palsy with otalgia and vesicular rash affecting the ear, may lead to hearing loss, reactivation of herpes zoster, acyclovir with steroids.

Seizures — focal: One part of the brain affected, aware or impaired awareness, motor symptoms (jerking, twitching, automatisms).

Seizures — generalised: All of the body so there is loss of consciousness, tonic-clonic (stiff then shake), and absence.

Sheehan's syndrome: Pituitary dysfunction after a postpartum haemorrhage (amenorrhoea or no lactation).

Somatisation disorder: **L**ots of **S**ymptoms, different body systems, almost always normal investigations.

Status epilepticus management: 1. A-E, intravenous lorazepam 4mg/Buccal Midazolam/Rectal Diazepam. 2. IV Phenytoin. 3. Anaesthetic input/phenobarbital.

Stroke mimics: 4 S's: **S**eizures, **S**epsis, **S**yncope, **S**ugar (hypoglycaemia).

Sturge-Weber syndrome: Facial port wine stain and eye problems.

Subacute sclerosing panencephalitis: Young child or adolescent, intellectual decline after measles infection, fatal.

Subarachnoid haemorrhage: Thunderclap headache, risk factors include hypertension and polycystic kidney disease, caused by aneurysms and trauma.

Subdural haematoma (acute): Falling or head injury, concave hyperdensity that crosses suture lines on CT scan, elderly and alcohol abuse risk factors.

Subdural haematoma (chronic): Trivial head injury, fluctuating consciousness level, concave hypodensity on CT scan.

Short-lasting, unilateral, neuralgiform headache attacks with conjunctival injection and tearing (SUNCT): Trigeminal autonomic cephalgia, headache happens hundreds of times a day, lasts seconds to minutes.

Syringomyelia: Central canal cerebrospinal fluid cavity, loss of pain and temperature in 'cape' distribution, hand muscle wasting, associated with Chiari malformations.

Tardive dyskinesia: Involuntary movements affecting the face, tongue, and mouth — caused by long-term antipsychotic use.

Temporal arteritis: See giant cell arteritis.

Thrombolysis criteria: <4.5 hours after symptoms, no contraindications (pregnancy, stroke in the last month, high blood pressure, no bleed on scan).

Todd's paresis: Weakness after a seizure, mimics a stroke.

Toxoplasmosis (cerebral): Fever, confusion, CNS signs — parasitic infection in immunocompromised patients!

Transverse myelitis: Inflammation of spinal cord with loss of function — think multiple sclerosis!

Trigeminal neuralgia: Fifth cranial nerve compression, sharp stabbing pain on the cheek resembling a toothache, worse by wind and touch, carbamazepine as first line treatment.

<u>Tuberous sclerosis</u>: Triad of intellectual disability, intractable epilepsy, and facial angiofibromas (adenoma sebaceum) — also presents with ash leaf macules and Shagreen patch on back.

<u>Vestibular schwannoma (acoustic neuroma)</u>: Schwann cell tumour, unilateral sensory hearing loss (cranial nerve VIII) with additional fifth and seventh cranial nerve involvement; think neurofibromatosis type 2 if bilateral!

<u>Weber's syndrome</u>: Third cranial nerve palsy and contralateral hemiplegia, midbrain infarct or lesion.

<u>Wernicke's (receptive) aphasia</u>: Temporal lobe, patient talks fluently but words make no sense!

<u>Wernicke's encephalopathy</u>: Acute vitamin B1 deficiency, triad of confusion, ataxia, and ophthalmoplegia.

<u>Wilson's disease</u>: Autosomal recessive disorder of copper metabolism, psychiatric disturbance in children, Kayser-Fleischer ring around the eye.

Index

CPSIA information can be obtained
at www.ICGtesting.com
Printed in the USA
JSHW022152141022
31669JS00002B/58